What people are saying about …

Just Show Up

"Kara Tippetts changed my life and thousands of others' lives because she was a rare, singular voice who, when facing the end of her life here, had street cred to speak about what really matters. Open these rich, radical pages and give yourself the gift of friendship like you've always wanted and community like you've only hoped for—before it's too late to *just show up*."

Ann Voskamp, *New York Times* bestselling
author of *One Thousand Gifts: A Dare
to Live Fully Right Where You Are*

Praise for …

The Hardest Peace

"Kara writes honestly about a subject that few of us want to confront. She even manages to find humor in the midst of a horrifying situation. Most importantly, she points readers to the hope that is found in a God whose grace is sufficient for every trial, and whose love for His children is steadfast even in the face of despair."

Jim Daly, president of Focus on the Family

"Kara Tippetts's book *The Hardest Peace* is at the same time deeply convicting and encouraging. Kara is brutally honest in sharing her struggles all the way from a young girl to now as a mother of four battling recurrent cancer. Through it all, she has found the deep reality of God's grace and love. This is a book everyone ought to read."

Jerry Bridges, author of *Trusting God: Even When Life Hurts*

"No one chooses suffering, but everyone has the freedom to choose how to respond to it. Because she chooses Christ, Kara Tippetts can not only endure the pain and ugliness of her pilgrimage through the desert of cancer, but on the journey, she can also find beauty, wonder, joy, and even freedom from the cares of this world. By showing us how to die, Kara Tippetts shows us how to live."

Rod Dreher, author of *The Little Way of Ruthie Leming*

"Losing myself in the startling light of Kara's story, I have found who I am, who He is, and more of the meaning of every breath."

Ann Voskamp, *New York Times* bestselling author of *One Thousand Gifts* justshowup

justshowup

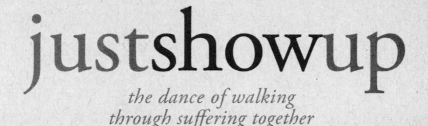

*the dance of walking
through suffering together*

kara tippetts

jill lynn buteyn

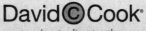

David C Cook®

transforming lives together

JUST SHOW UP
Published by David C Cook
4050 Lee Vance View
Colorado Springs, CO 80918 U.S.A.

David C Cook Distribution Canada
55 Woodslee Avenue, Paris, Ontario, Canada N3L 3E5

David C Cook U.K., Kingsway Communications
Eastbourne, East Sussex BN23 6NT, England

The graphic circle C logo is a registered trademark of David C Cook.

The website addresses recommended throughout this book are offered as a
resource to you. These websites are not intended in any way to be or imply an
endorsement on the part of David C Cook, nor do we vouch for their content.

All Scripture quotations are taken from the Holy Bible, New International
Version®, NIV®. Copyright © 1973, 2011 by Biblica, Inc.® Used by permission
of Zondervan. All rights reserved worldwide. www.zondervan.com.

LCCN 2015936252
ISBN 978-1-4347-0953-0
eISBN 978-1-4347-0961-5

Published in association with William K. Jensen Literary
Agency, 119 Bampton Court, Eugene, OR 97404

The Team: Ingrid Beck, John Blase, Nick Lee, Helen Macdonald, Karen Athen
Cover Design: Amy Konyndyk
Cover Photo: istockphoto.com

Printed in the United States of America
First Edition 2015

2 3 4 5 6 7 8 9 10

082815

Contents

Introduction   9

Chapter 1 — The Value of Showing Up   13

Chapter 2 — The Dance of Showing Up   33

Chapter 3 — The Gift of Silence   51

Chapter 4 — The Nurturing of Friendships   77

Chapter 5 — The Art of Giving and Receiving   95

Chapter 6 — The Battle of Insecurity   115

Chapter 7 — The Highs and Lows Together   135

Chapter 8 — The Future Plans   155

Chapter 9 — The Beauty of Community   175

Introduction

You have to be grateful whenever you get to someplace safe and okay, even if it turns out it wasn't quite where you were heading.

Anne Lamott, *Small Victories*

Hi. My name is Kara Tippetts, and I may not be alive when you read this book. I hope so, but I don't know. That decision is in the hands of the Author of my life—His name is Jesus. I trust Him with every ounce of who I am. The reality is I am dying, and some of that story is told in my book *The Hardest Peace*. There are other pieces that were hinted at in that book but not developed at length. It's not because those pieces aren't important, because they are. It's just that they were best kept for another book, one that I hoped to write with my good friend Jill.

Jill and I dreamed and talked about writing a book together, one that would try to take the mystery out of walking with one another through suffering. That's the book you have in your hands. We would have liked to write a book that took the uncomfortable or awkward out, but there's no way we could do that and be honest. Because honestly, it's hard. But it's not difficult. You just have to show up. That's not some kind of secret figurative language. We're talking about literally showing up.

There is so much power in showing up, humble power in saying, "I'm here. I may not have the answers, but I'm here." Most often it's those who come without answers or agendas who are the most helpful. Those people have been invaluable to our home. Jill has been one of those people. That's why I wanted her help on this project. She knows what she's writing about. In being a friend to me during this season, she's seen the bad, the ugly, and the horrible. But she's also seen the beautiful. And the beautiful has been worth it. So worth it.

Life can be numbing when the story is flailing along in suffering. Life can be pretty difficult even on the good days, but throw cancer or divorce or bankruptcy or the death of a child into the mix and everything becomes dizzying. Sometimes even paralyzing. So often we would be spinning in weariness from my latest diagnosis or round of tests and we'd even forget to eat. Can you imagine, forgetting to eat? It's true. But the sensitive hearts of our community showed up, ready to help.

It has been beautiful to watch God gently care for our needs so specifically through the care of our community. The care came in both unexpected and specific ways most days. Ways that I didn't ask for or know I needed. But even more than my needs, God has cared for the tender hearts of my children and my husband. He has shepherded and protected them fiercely throughout my diagnosis, and now as we are moving toward my last breath, I see the gentle hand of protection ever upon my family, ready with present grace to walk them through the hard good-bye.

In my affliction, as I see more hard come, I know we will be kept. I often say my story is one that has been shattered into a million pieces but that each piece is known and loved. The shattered pieces of us all are known, intimately known. As I see our community surround us, I see the intimate knowing of God in our situation. Showing up for another says, "I see you. Your pain is known, and though I cannot make it better, I'm here and that's what matters." Showing up for another, extending yourself for another, is always costly. Always. So why do it? There are several reasons, actually, that we'll cover in this book. But one of the most important is community. Another way to say that is "friends."

I no longer call you servants, because a servant does not know his master's business. Instead, I have called you friends, for everything that I learned from my Father I have made known to you.

John 15:15

Friends. Community. It is the only way to know and be known. It's where we see our own humanity and frailty, our gifts and our weaknesses. When we show up for one another, we invade each other in love and become witnesses to the truth that trials and sickness and pain are not the whole story. There's more, so much more. We can remind one another that our lives are not a mistake. And, most importantly, that we are loved with an everlasting love.

Editor's note: Kara Tippetts went home to Jesus on March 22, 2015, after a long battle with breast cancer. Kara completed her contributions to this book before her death. Therefore her words carry the tone of the present tense, as they should.

Chapter 1

The Value of Showing Up

Your heart is riding around in my backyard on a trike and I want to weep. Okay, I did a little while making the mac n' cheese and reading your last blog. But I wiped up those tears before the littles came upstairs. I feel as though I sit on the fringe of your cancer. We are moms together. I know no other way to describe my heart. I think the reason complete strangers read your blog and feel like they know you is because you lay it all on the line. Your heart is completely open. In the good and the bad. You let people in. It's a gift.

You have counseled me with wisdom on the playground while our children play and swing. We quickly moved past pretending into some great conversations.

We might not have years between us, but we are friends.

We are moms together. And that's why all of this matters so much.

In my midtwenties, I had my first real encounter with suffering. Before that time, I didn't really know or understand hard. I certainly didn't know it could be used as a noun until Kara.

I had experienced small things in life that felt like enormous problems, but nothing shook my world until I had my first baby. She had colic and cried much of the day and night. I spent hours feeding, holding, and walking with her, attempting to comfort her while she was in obvious pain. But nothing seemed to work.

Certainly there are many worse hardships, but this became the thing that rocked my previously mundane life. I was a young mom feeling completely alone, helpless, and depressed.

I did attempt to reach out to some people, but it took so much effort that holing up was easier. While Kara is an extrovert and a gatherer of people, I am an introvert. I love people but refuel alone. During the time we were dealing with colic, I began to hide. I lacked the energy to do more than survive.

While doctors do what they can for colic, they also nudge you out the door and tell you it will pass. I was told to hang on, that my child would grow out of it.

I hung on by my fingernails, dangling from the side of a cliff.

I know numerous people showed up for me during that period, but I specifically remember one friend. I didn't want her to come over. Remember, I'm an introvert (text, don't call) and I prefer to enjoy my misery alone.

She came anyway.

She brought lunch and we sat at the kitchen table. She didn't remark on my appearance, though I'm guessing it wasn't a shining moment for me. Nor did she comment on the fact that I clutched my daughter to my chest and never offered to let her hold the baby. That would have been a logical decision on my part, but I was nowhere near normal functioning at that moment.

I don't remember any particulars of the conversation we had. That part didn't really matter. I do remember the microwave beeping once a minute to remind me that I'd reheated my coffee for the thousandth time. I didn't get up to stop it. Not once did my friend mention this annoying sound.

Why didn't I move from my chair and stop the beeping? I don't know. I know only that even if I wasn't physically paralyzed in that moment of my life, I was stuck. I couldn't function.

My friend wasn't afraid to push into my messy life and simply sit with me. We didn't spend hours together. In fact, the whole experience didn't last all that long. We ate. She made me keep the leftovers, and then she was gone.

She showed up.

She didn't pester me about why I was so crazy to not let someone else hold my child. She didn't try to fix me or even advise me. She was simply soft in a place that felt like broken glass. I'll never forget her showing up, though I don't remember what was said.

Showing up is not a new concept, but sometimes it feels that way. Something in our culture has told us to pull back, to protect ourselves from hurt, from people, from entering in with one another.

And there's a reason for that. Showing up can get us hurt in the biggest ways. People disappoint and wound us. Or, in the case of walking through suffering with a friend or loved one, it can hurt beyond anything we've ever imagined. Take-me-out-at-the-knees, ugly-cry hurt.

As I write this, Kara is in a lot of pain. While I can pray and beg for relief for her, I have nothing in my arsenal for helping with pain relief. I want to make it better. I like to fix things. But I can't fix this. I can't change the fact that, barring a miracle, her babies are going to be without a mother one day. Or that her husband has an unimaginably hard journey to walk when she leaves this earth.

And that's painful.

So, yeah, showing up isn't easy at times.

But maybe that's why there's such value to be found in it. I've learned real beauty lies in the good that comes out of the hard. While walking through suffering with a friend or loved one can hurt in the biggest ways, it also brings the greatest blessings. It changes people. Showing up can be the greatest gift ever given or received.

The *New York Times* bestseller *The Purpose-Driven Life* has a first line I will never forget.

It's not about you.

As I thought about how to walk artfully through suffering with a friend or loved one, that phrase kept swimming through my mind. It's true. As a friend in this journey, it really isn't about me.

This just makes sense. I can't fix my friend's suffering, so when there's an opportunity to help, I want to help. But at the same time, the relationship can feel skewed. There's no more even stephen. The balance is rocked.

Consistently the relationship will become about the person suffering, purely because that is how it has to be.

Except in the same way, this journey is not even about the one suffering.

For Kara, it might feel like it is when meals are being brought to her home or someone else is doing the laundry that will clothe her children. But she's letting people help—not because that's the easy choice, but because it's not about her.

Kara would rather be the one giving to a friend, the one serving, the one doing laundry love for her family. But many times through this journey, she has been physically unable to do those things.

Walking through suffering with a loved one strips the pretense away. Kara cannot be all things to her family. But she could grind her feet into the ground and refuse to accept help. It's not about her in the same way that my journey has become not about me.

And that's where God enters the picture and it becomes all about Him.

How does He want me to show up? What's my role according to Him? Will I accept the role God has asked of me even when it's not the one I wanted?

Kara has had to answer those same questions as she's walked her side of this.

That's why she's written a blog and a book and has been so beautifully honest about her journey. When God prompted her to share her hard and her heart with others, she listened.

Each of Kara's friends has worked to do the same in what God has asked of them. For some, it's been not being able to be physically present with Kara. They are in other states and not close to her, even though being close is exactly where they want to be. I've watched so many of them accept this and decide to walk this journey from afar without grumbling, though their hearts are hurting beyond comprehension.

One friend told me that she was feeling sorry for herself, frustrated that she couldn't be close by to help. Then she realized she did have a way to honor Kara from a distance.

She decided to love her own children and husband with the kind of big love Kara so freely gives. It isn't her first choice to be unable to physically help with needs, but she's obeying.

Another group of families have become caregivers of the children. Their children match in ages and their homes have become safe havens for the kids. Another mom's gifting is in making meals for the freezer. The list goes on and on.

We might not feel qualified to show up. I know I never have and probably never will. But God uses those of us who aren't qualified so that He's glorified.

And when we show up, we're blessed.

I first met Kara when she and her family moved to Colorado to plant a church. My husband, kids, and I went to the church that their plant sprouted from. Our kids went to the same school, and our daughters were in the same class.

They showed up in the middle of the school year, and that summer she was diagnosed with breast cancer.

Six months isn't a lot of time to forge a friendship. I think we both liked each other, but there was no rush to share halved matching heart necklaces. She and Jason were easy, and I thought we had time. Time to choose each other in health. Time for our kids to grow up together and a friendship to develop.

Once her diagnosis came, I remember thinking, *We haven't been friends long enough for this. I haven't known her that long, so now what?*

I didn't know if I fit, or where I fit. We'd done only that dance of interest, the one that says, *Hmm, I like her. I think we could be friends. She's sarcastic enough, so there's that connection. Yeah, let's see what happens.*

But in the crushing blow of her cancer diagnosis, everything changed.

Suddenly *Let's see what happens* became *Either you're in or you're out.* It wasn't a mandate put out by Kara or anything crazy like that. It was just a movement, a sense that there was a decision to be made regarding this friendship.

Despite not knowing where I fit or what was to come, I distinctly remember the process of choosing to enter in with her.

Now I see that the Holy Spirit was nudging me to show up, but back then I simply felt pulled toward Kara. Connected because of our littles.

Other friends felt there was a choice to be made too. And in those moments, many of us decided to walk this journey with the Tippetts family. In a way, I think we all committed to stumbling together, knowing trials were coming and things were not going to be easy.

Little did we know how hard it was going to get.

But for me, more doubts loomed than just navigating the beginnings of a friendship. I had never walked through hard with a friend before. At least, not walked well. What if I didn't know what to say to Kara and Jason, or said the wrong thing? What if I offended them or said something stupid? (That last one was a very real possibility. I tend to trip a lot in life, physically and verbally.)

In that diagnosis, Jason and Kara went from easy to not so easy. I didn't have a clue how to do suffering with a friend.

With those doubts still swirling in my mind, I took a step off the edge of a cliff. Or maybe God gave me a little push.

Many times when Kara would blog about how cancer was affecting her life, I would write answers expressing my feelings. I would save them on my computer, but I wouldn't hit publish. There was nowhere for those words to go—they didn't fit on my blog—but I had to write to purge my soul of all the feelings her journey invoked.

These writings are what you see at the beginning of my parts of the book, my thoughts from along the way.

As you can see from what you've already read, my journey with Kara—my attempts to figure out how to show up and why I felt called to show up—started with this one phrase:

We are mothers together.

In the strange dance between feeling as though we hadn't been friends long enough and the tug that prompted me to show up, I kept coming back to this one conclusion.

We are mothers together.

That's where I started my journey of showing up.

One day, I was upset about my daughter, worried about a medical problem that has since been resolved. Things like that tend to consume me, and I can be a worrier of the worst sort. I couldn't get my mind off the *what ifs* regarding what was going on with my daughter.

That same day Kara was going into a chemo treatment, something that always took a lot out of her. She would get sick for days and days, and could hardly keep anything down. She'd just blogged about how she wasn't able to do the errands she used to be able to, and so I texted her.

"What can I do for you? I know there's something. Give me something."

Her reply came back that after each chemo treatment, she chose a new drink to try to stay hydrated. Because she threw up so much, she didn't want the same thing as the last time. She gave me a few suggestions of things that sounded good and then asked if I could drop off some new choices for her.

I went a little overboard in the drink aisle. But in helping her, I forgot my fears for my daughter. They subsided, their edges rounded out by peace.

I stopped thinking about myself, and it made all the difference.

Kara could have told me she was fine when I texted her. She could have asked Jason or another one of her close friends to get drinks for her.

But she let me in.

Showing up in suffering benefits both sides, and it has to be entered in from both sides.

Had she pushed me away or continuously not accepted my offers of help, our relationship would not be what it is today.

I didn't fully recognize the value in showing up until I was pulled into this journey.

I was afraid of doing the wrong thing, and I didn't have a clue where to begin. But when we step out in the middle of our fear, God meets us there.

I can honestly say for myself—and for any friend I've talked to—there are no regrets about showing up.

Kara has recently been moved to hospice care. Our tears, pain, questions, and fears are numerous right now. We are messy in our suffering.

But we are messy together.

If you're peeking in the window and seeing only heartbreak, then you're missing the bigger picture.

Open the doors wide so that you can see the community that has been built during this hard journey. The friendships formed. The modeling of doing life together that has changed people's lives.

Faith and community have sprouted and flourished. Deeper relationships have grown. We all have to depend on Him. On each other.

Fear is a lonely companion.

Look what I would have missed had I let those whispers of doubts win.

It would have been a lonely existence if I had hid myself away, worrying about saying or doing the wrong thing, or if I had held back because Kara and I didn't have a friendship that spanned years. This experience has changed me for the rest of my life.

Yes, I've been stretched in places that don't feel good as I watch cancer eat away at my friend. But while my soul might be writhing in that pain, something beautiful has come from the pushing and pulling and discomfort.

I've grown. I've learned so much from Kara and from doing friendship during her suffering.

I no longer feel like that person I once was.

I still struggle in certain areas, but I feel as though I've shed one layer of me so another could be revealed. Another step on the path to doing what God asks of me.

Right now, it's hard. Harder than hard. But would I go back to the person I once was? If I could fly away to that moment of choosing Kara, of entering in, would I choose differently?

No. This is a journey we're meant to walk together. The joys, the hurt, the grace that always shows up, and the beauty God orchestrates when we show up for each other are amazing to see.

It might be scary, but this is where God wants us. In the trenches, getting our clothes dirty, and stumbling to figure out community here on earth.

I would never go back.

This might be harder than I ever imagined it would be, but I meant these words I recently texted to Kara:

> I'm writing about meeting you. About choosing to enter into a relationship, knowing it could be hard. About how I've never regretted that decision, though along the way bad news sent me sobbing to the floor of my house on more than one occasion. I would choose you all over again, Kara. You've changed my life, and the journey together has changed my life. And that's what this book is about for me. Big love. People are missing out when they don't enter the lives of those around them.

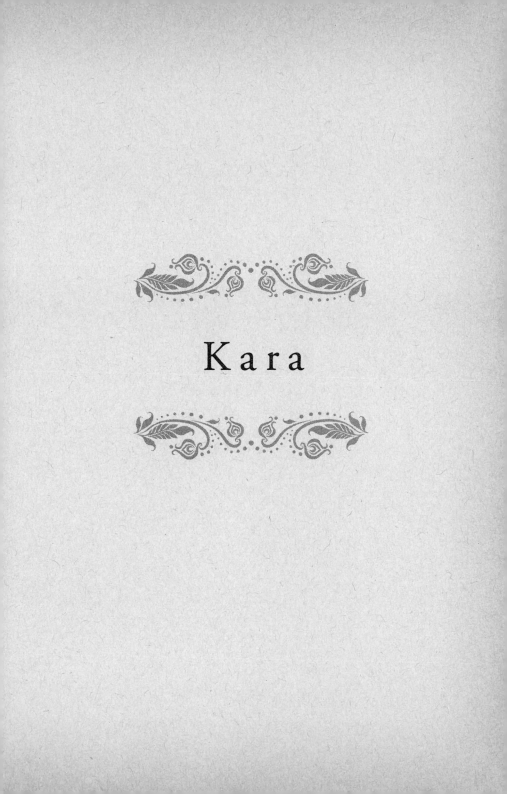

Kara

The other day my editor asked me if I was familiar with *The Four Loves* by C. S. Lewis. I said, *"Oh no, should I be?"* He laughed and then went on to list them: affection, brotherly love, romance, and God-love. We talked for a few minutes about each one, after which I said, *"That all makes perfect sense, but I simply prefer big love."* He laughed again.

Big love. It's one of my favorite phrases. It's really the only way I know how to love. And it's certainly become more focused since my initial diagnosis. Like Jill said, my time is limited. So I'm trying to squeeze every drop of life out of every day, because like that movie tries to tell us every year at Christmas, *it really is a wonderful life.* I don't know how much more time I have. But the truth is, none of us do. Open any newspaper, turn on any news broadcast, check what's trending online and I promise you you'll find a story about someone who was here yesterday but is not here today. Whatever time they thought they had was just that—a thought.

It's sad to me that most of us don't practice big love until something tragic enters our lives. To try to remedy that, the common challenge we hear is "Live like today is your last day." That's not bad advice, but I just don't think it always works unless there is something like cancer to give that phrase some teeth. I think a better approach is "Live like today is your very first day." Think about that for a minute. What if you and I lived today like it was a fresh start, like we got a do-over and could start showing up and practicing big love from the very beginning? Can you imagine the impact on our families, our friendships, our churches?

Each chapter will conclude with two questions designed to help you start showing up. If you're reading through the book on your own, write out your answers in the margins or somewhere on the page (it's your book after all). If you happen to be working through this book with a friend or a group, use these questions as discussion prompts for the times you get together. The goal is not to give perfect answers, but honest ones.

1. The first step in showing up is answering the question, *Who?* Who do you know who is currently suffering and you want or need to show up for? You may know right away. Then again, you may not be sure. If it's not clear, ask God to bring that person's name or face to your thoughts, and trust your thoughts when they come.

2. Once you've got that person's face in mind, what fears or anxieties do you have about showing up for them? You may not have a long list, but there will always be one or two. It's a good idea to write those down or share them with a trusted friend. The most important thing at the outset is to name those fears because that takes away some of their power.

Chapter 2

The Dance of Showing Up

Another text from Kara. This one makes me well up. Most of them do. It sounds bad. That is all I know. Jason isn't home to be with Kara at this appointment. Someone needs to go with her. No one should go through this alone. I miss her phone call, and the rest of the day I wonder, Did someone go? Is she okay? Of course she's not okay. But is there someone there during the not okay? Who has the kids? I take a deep breath. She would tell me if she needed me. She would ask. I know this. I try to breathe again, try to go about my house doing laundry and putting dishes in the dishwasher as if my friend isn't hearing a diagnosis that will change the course of her life. She's constantly on my mind. I don't hear specific news after her appointment, but I don't need to. Not until she's ready. I know she's processing, waiting for Jason to get back from his trip. In the evening I get a text, but it's not about the appointment or what the doctor said. It's about writing.

"I still want to write our book."

"Me too," I answer, and her text back makes me laugh so loud the kids ask what I'm laughing about.

"But will you hit publish?"

Kara knows I write things all the time that I don't post. I probably wouldn't have sent in my fiction work if God hadn't orchestrated that. Is it the fear of failure? Yes. But it's also the need for privacy. I write everything down—my brain won't stop until it's processed on paper—and yet, most of the time, I don't hit publish. Sometimes it's just too personal, too raw. Will people understand me questioning God yet trusting Him at the same time?

I wake around six thirty the next morning, and my first thought is of Kara. Lord, I whisper. It's the only prayer I have right now. Lord. I just keep saying His name. And it is a prayer, but I don't even know what I am asking for. Peace? Wisdom? A different life for my friend? Yet it's not a diagnosis I need. I don't want to hear where the cancer has gone. Just typing that sentence brings a rush of moisture to my eyes. What I need to know is if she's okay. Has she gone to the dark place to mourn and cry and rage that this shouldn't be her life? That's where I would be. But Kara almost always surprises me. Today there will probably be a blog post, and she might state things are not well, but she always, always comes back to Jesus. How can a person not be attracted to that kind of friendship?

In twelve years of marriage, Corrie has spent a total of five years apart from her husband. It hasn't been all at once, but over the course of several deployments and overseas positions, she has taken care of their three little girls and has run the household.

While she is one of the most capable people I've ever met, everyone needs a support team. When I asked Corrie if anyone ever showed up for her, she said yes. One particular person impressed her the most.

During a year when Corrie's husband was gone, a woman came up to her at church and asked Corrie if her daughters could use another grandparent. The woman said she wanted to show up at Corrie's house once a week and be there so that Corrie could accomplish whatever she needed to do.

Corrie responded, *"How about Wednesday?"*

This woman and this offer amaze me, but what struck me even more were Corrie's next words.

"So many people offer to help. They say, let me know if you need anything, but that offer is easily dismissed because it's too broad."

I cringed because I've said that same thing to people more times than I can count. Even worse, I remember saying those exact words to Corrie.

I knew with her husband overseas that Corrie had a lot on her shoulders. My offer of "Let me know if you need anything" was legitimate. I meant it. But now I see it through her eyes. That is a broad offer. What did I expect her to say?

I think back through those days, and I imagine simple things that could have helped.

Her house was on my way home. I could have offered to drop the girls off after school. I could have been better about offering rides to birthday parties or taking them for playdates. The list of things I could have suggested is long. But I didn't know that specifics made all the difference in showing up for someone. I wanted to help—I was willing. I just didn't know how.

For many of us, the desire to help is strong. We feel that tug, the prompting from the Holy Spirit. We long to do something concrete that takes stress away, even if it's a small something.

The beauty in offering a specific help instead of a broad one is that we get to help within our gifting.

This concept makes me a little giddy because taking people a meal stresses me out. Yet I've always struggled to do it anyway. The idea that I can listen to the Holy Spirit and then offer within the gifts He's given me is freeing.

When I had babies, people brought me some pretty glorious meals. In comparison, the red-in-the-face, slightly panicked version of me that shows up on a front step when I take a meal isn't pretty. And the meal probably isn't very spectacular either.

Don't get me wrong. I love, LOVE when people bring me a meal. Preferably one with something wrapped in bacon. But I do think some people are gifted in this area. When I do accomplish taking a meal to someone, I can guarantee I don't have anything ready for my family when I get back home. We usually end up having to grab something.

Sometimes a meal is the only way to help, and in those instances I've come up with a plan to take away my panic. I have a go-to meal. Something already planned out that I can do every time and that's comfortable for me. It can even be premade. For me, it's usually an entrée from the deli at Costco. Add a bag of salad, and that's about as gourmet as it gets around here.

Maybe you don't even have that in you. Perhaps a gift card is your go-to dinner. I wouldn't complain if that were the case. Would you?

Sometimes we just have to accept our gifting. Or lack of gifting.

And there is freedom in knowing that God made us just the way we are for a reason. That maybe the thing we do well is exactly what our friend or loved one needs.

We put so much pressure on ourselves to do everything right that many of us decide it's too hard to even attempt entering into someone else's suffering.

The beauty in showing up, in choosing to enter the dance even though you might not know the steps, is that God creates something beautiful from our attempts.

The more you do something, the easier it gets. Showing up is the same.

And after you decide to attend the party, your moves will get better and your decisions will feel more natural.

Doubt, second-guessing, and confusion will still be your companions for much of the journey, though they should lessen the further you enter in.

I've known Kara for about three years. She's had cancer for two and a half of those. I've come a long way from when I first started showing up for her, but I still struggle with doubts of what to do.

Kara's wise friend Ruth calls it *the tension*.

That visual beautifully describes what is felt as we walk through suffering with someone and make decisions regarding how to show up. We're pulled in two directions, or six directions, and we don't know which way is right.

How am I supposed to help? How do I show up? Does showing up mean staying away? Did that last sentence even make sense?

This week Kara learned there are no more medical options for her to fight cancer with, and she's being moved to a hospice care team. It's been three days since she heard the news. It feels like so little time to process, yet everything moves at hyperspeed. There's less time to question and wonder because opportunities feel as though they could slip through our fingers.

I wonder if I'll get to hug her one last time. Do we have days? Weeks? Months? She doesn't even know the answer to that question, and it's her life, her body.

The answer rests in God's hands, and His only.

Tonight, another friend and I did the dance regarding how we should show up for Kara. We didn't know if we should go visit. In these moments, it's hard to know whether we are a help or a bother. Whether seeing her is about encouraging her or filling a need of our own.

During a twenty-minute phone conversation—unfortunately true, but many times we've just had to hash out our doubts and concerns with a friend—we worked through some questions. Who is this friend of ours? She's an extrovert. She refuels with people. They give her energy. Because I'm an introvert, the thought of wanting people around me if I were suffering, or had received news like Kara had, just seems foreign. I would be curled into a ball with a No Visitors sign hanging from my door.

But that's not our girl.

As the two of us girlfriends overanalyzed, we also asked, what is God asking of us? This one is harder to decipher, and so we prayed He would guide us.

We love our Kara, and outside of all this cancer muck, she is our girlfriend. The one we've laughed and cried with and would give anything to continue living life with.

The one whose children we've committed to loving.

We believed showing up would show her how important she is to us, and so we finally decided to go see her.

Did we make the right decision? I'm still not sure. We felt relief and peace in seeing her, and we hope it was the right decision. But there will be times while walking through suffering and trials with others when even after you've made a choice, you won't know if you made the right one.

Many times the answers won't be clear-cut.

We'd like specific directions for showing up. But it's not so simple. Every decision depends on the prompting of the Holy Spirit.

Pray for wisdom. Seek guidance.

And at times, even though we have the best intentions, mistakes will be made. That's just the nature of this dance.

You'll need to have grace for and with each other. Lots and lots of it.

Grace is the glue that holds relationships together as we walk through suffering with one another.

As we make decisions on how best to show up, we're also going to need our flexibility capes. What works one time might not be the answer the next time.

I'm not very good with that *flexibility* word. I prefer concrete details. But God is constantly reminding me some things are mine to hold not with an iron grip, but with open hands.

That's what this book has become for me. Another question: What does God have in store? Does He want me to keep writing?

Or does He want me to let go of the dream of writing this book with Kara?

When the contract for this book first came through, Kara had just entered the hospital for the first time. The medicine affected her so strongly I didn't know if this book was a possibility. I knew I could write from a friend's perspective, but what about Kara's part? She's so wise. I learn from her every time I talk to her. She has a gift of speaking into people's lives. It's part of why we all love her so much.

When I went to see Kara tonight, I was stuck in these unknowns, unable to see a clear path. What would come of our writing? Could it still happen? What would God do with it? Kara and I have dreamed about this book together. Not writing it seems impossible. Writing it seems impossible. I'm so broken by Kara's news that putting the book aside seems like the only option.

Kara's friend Ruth sensed my unease and gently asked me questions. Then she imparted this bit of wisdom:

"It's okay to tell God you don't know where to go from here."

Relief coursed through me at the needed reminder that God is not surprised by my lack of knowledge or direction.

It's okay to not know if I'm supposed to write or not. *It's okay* to be not okay. Lost and broken is God's specialty.

It's okay to not know how to show up for someone or how to take the first steps into walking through suffering with a friend.

Ask for guidance. He will meet you there.

You can tell Him how you feel and what your fears are, and He will open the path for you to take a first step. And then the step after that.

The tension of not knowing what to do will stay with you as you show up for each other. And it will create a dependence on God and the community around you instead of on yourself.

With the news that Kara is being moved to hospice care, it's stressful right now. The illusion of time we've all been clinging to has been shattered. People across the country are asking if they should come, how they can help. The tension of how to show up is being felt by many.

One friend wanted to come, but she didn't know when she should or how best to show up. Kara and Jason are being bombarded by offers of help—on top of dealing with this unfathomable situation—and they don't have the ability to answer everyone or make all those decisions.

After this friend prayed about it and sought counsel, someone advised her to stop asking the ones suffering to make a decision. Instead, she made plans, finding her own transportation and a place to stay outside of Jason and Kara's home. Then she told them, *"I'm coming and I'd love to see you. But if it doesn't work out, I understand."*

I feel like we need to pause and have a *Saved by the Bell* time-out moment right now. I am not saying to disregard what someone says, jump in a car, and throw yourself into the person's life. If they say no or not right now, respect their answers.

This friend didn't show up on Jason and Kara's doorstep with a suitcase. She knew she might not see Kara at all. What a humbling thing to do. When I would want details and commitments, she went openhanded. It wasn't about her. She wanted to be available to them if they needed her, but she knew the answer might be no when she showed up.

She said when she stopped laying the burden of that decision on them, she had peace—even without knowing what the outcome would be once she arrived.

After her plans were made, Jason and Kara were able to respond more easily about their part in them. They were no longer being asked to make the decision. And she'd given them freedom from her expectations.

The one time I did attempt to take a meal to Kara's family, I was running late because of bad traffic, and I didn't get to their house until the kids were hungry and ready for dinner to be on the table. Thank goodness it was hot and ready to go. I remember wanting to scramble out of their house as fast as possible. It was dinnertime. I wanted to let them eat. My kids turn into crazy monsters when they are hungry, as do I.

I'll never forget Jason's face by the front door when he told me Kara was too sick to see me, that she was resting.

Of course, was my first thought. I hadn't expected to see Kara.

But Jason didn't know that.

Kara's been too ill most of the time to see the people who take meals to her family. I know this is hard for her. Of course she wants to thank each person who slaved over a meal for her family. (I say "slaved" because that's how it feels to me. And also, after this book comes out, no one's going to accept dinner from me ever again. I should feel worse about that than I do.)

Your person might want to see you and say thank you, but they may be physically unable. Maybe they are sleeping for the first time all day. Maybe they can't muster the strength—whether physical or emotional—to see another person outside of their immediate family.

If we go and serve not expecting to see them, even telling the family we're not asking for their time, that is another gift we can give. Drop the meal off, do the laundry, or pick up the kids without expectations. People are going to welcome you when you want to serve and you aren't making it about you.

This can be tough because sometimes we just miss our people. We want to see them. I get it. I really do. I'm tearing up writing these words because while walking through suffering with someone brings a lot of blessings, there will be times when you'll mourn the way a relationship once was. Suffering can steal friendship moments from us—ones we really want to keep having. We crave those same conversations we used to have and the time we used to spend together.

But suffering changes things. And another way to love your person is to release expectations that would remain with a normal friendship. Kara always talks about finding a new normal. That's exactly what you'll need to look for. And while missing your person and the way things used to be is hard, there's peace when your actions aren't wrapped up in your personal agendas.

I wish I could tell you I'm writing this book because I've done so much right during this journey, but if anything, it's the opposite. That's why it's a dance of showing up. We're going to make mistakes, step on toes. But the good news is we mean well. We're showing up out of love, and that does come across to the person suffering.

God will have a plan in your showing up. You might play a small role, or your role could be large. But He wants you there for a reason, even if that reason is just to learn dependence on Him.

Whatever you do, don't get overwhelmed and quit dancing. Just like Kara, I love to dance, even if I look like a fool doing it. Showing up, even if you make mistakes, will still bless you and the person suffering far beyond anything you've ever imagined.

This book isn't about doing it perfectly. It's about doing it better together.

Kara

I love to dance. But you know what I love even more than dancing? Watching my kids jump around like crazy to the beat of one of our favorite songs. Their bodies give way to the rhythm of the music and all I see is innocence and energy and passion. They don't necessarily know what the steps are; they just feel the music and want to move. I love it! That's why dance is such a great image to keep in mind as we practice showing up. Jill's sentence is so true: *"It's okay to not know how to show up for someone or how to take the first steps into walking through suffering with a friend."*

For Christ's love compels us …
2 Corinthians 5:14

Our wanting to show up, even if we don't know what to do or say or even feel, comes because something is nudging us, or rather Someone. It's the love of Christ compelling us to not just sit there but to get up and move. To show up. And if we can keep that in mind—that Christ's love is what's tugging at our hearts—then it's never just Jill moving toward me on her own. It's always Jill and Jesus moving toward me. Or Jesus and me moving toward Jill. So when we say this book is about doing it better together, that word *together* means all of us, but at the very center is Jesus, Immanuel, God-with-us.

1. Next comes the question, *What?* What is it that you, specifically you, can offer to that person in terms of big love? Again, you may know right away. But if you don't, then don't worry. Ask God, "What are You asking of me?" Then you may have to spend a little time in their space to see a need or recognize a way that you can specifically invade their life with love.

2. When was the last time someone showed up for you during a crisis of some sort? Who was it, and what did they do? They may have fumbled a little or maybe even a lot, but they still showed up. Have you taken the time to thank them? Even if you have, consider sending a note or making a phone call or sending a text (smile, introverts!) to say something like, "Hey, thanks again for showing up for me! You didn't have to, but you did, and it mattered."

Chapter 3

The Gift of Silence

I went to the movie The Fault in Our Stars with Kara and a few other girlfriends, and I did not cry. Maybe two tears slipped out. I am the crier of all criers. I cry at commercials, books, a well-said sentence. But I sat down the row from my friend who's suffering from cancer, and I did not cry. Why? I don't know. I imagine I distanced myself from the story on the screen. I distanced myself from the types of cancers, the way they attack, the sneaky way they slither into different parts of the body. I did not cry, but I shook.

After the movie, we stayed. Sweet friends spoke so freely with one another. Each moment of life is open, able to be talked about. But not from me. I don't have words. Unless they are to steal a laugh. I wait for the moments of laughter, squeezing each one out when I can. My friends are truth speakers, and they do not hide. They openly speak of Kara dying, as does she. But I am hiding behind some grasp of hope, some something. Only here, with a keyboard in front of me, do I have words. Why? I imagine it is as Kara has said. Because we write, write, write. And somehow, this anonymity of saying to everyone is easier than saying to the close ones.

Yesterday I got a text from Kara with tough news. The tears were instant. Because this is my girl, this is her real story. And I cannot distance myself from that.

Kara and I should be friends later in life, I think. We haven't had enough time. To be with her through this, I should be a lifelong friend, an early friend. I shouldn't have entered her life in the last few years. And then I remember. These are the early years. We should still have the next twenty or thirty or forty left. This should be the beginning of watching our kids grow up together, graduate together. This should be the beginning! I scream at God. He simply listens. I wonder if He tires of my shoulds—as if I somehow know better than He does.

People continue to say that God is working in this, in Kara's story. I know this to be true, but I am weary of hearing it. Not because I don't believe, but because the journey is hard for my friend. The suffering Kara endures steals my breath. The fear she faces starts the tremors again. It's too much for one person to bear. I am not okay with this. I tell God over and over again.

He simply listens.

And today, this is the only truth I have.

Years ago, the pastor who baptized our daughter was diagnosed with ALS.

There was a time when he was no longer preaching but still attended church. Each Sunday he would sit at one of the tables in the lobby and I would walk by.

I didn't have the right words, so I didn't show up.

I was scared. Scared that if I attempted to talk to him, it would be uncomfortable. Worried that I'd make things awkward for him or me. I remember trying to smile, but even that felt empty. There's something about a terminal illness that steals our tongues and strikes fear in our hearts. We're paralyzed. Well, maybe you aren't, but I was.

I've always regretted my actions with him. What if I would have just sat down with him at the same table? Would he have needed conversation from me? Did he need me to fill the air with platitudes he already knew?

I'm guessing silence would have been fine.

When Kara's news first came, I remember thinking about that time with my beloved pastor. I didn't want to be afraid or act that way again. I knew I didn't have answers and that I would probably never know what to say. But I didn't want to treat Kara or Jason differently because of a diagnosis.

So I decided I would show up for them, even if I simply stood by them in silence.

Easier said than done.

When our loved ones are suffering, we so badly want to say the right thing. Preferably something wise, encouraging, and comforting at the same time. Perhaps a Bible verse we've memorized for moments such as this or something insightful to earn a bunch of likes on Facebook.

But our people are not expecting profound answers from us—they don't want them. Hard is hard. And a perfectly phrased thought isn't going to fix it.

I understand the desire to say something comforting. From the outside, we can feel helpless around our hurting loved ones. We're working to meet their physical needs. Saying the right thing feels like another way we can help. It often takes me five minutes to craft a response to a text containing tough news from Kara because I so badly want to offer her comfort.

One time, after receiving particularly bad news from Kara, I remember thinking, *I have to say something more than my usual "I don't know what to say."*

I'd been praying for hope, asking God to show up in all of this hard and give us good news.

So, in my brilliance, I texted this: *"I just keep praying for hope."*

Kara replied, *"We already have it. It just might not be in the way we want it."*

See how far my attempt at saying the right thing got me? My suffering friend ended up encouraging me.

In text or real conversation with Kara, I have rarely come up with anything beyond "This stinks. I'm sorry. I'm praying. I love you." In the hard we've walked through together as friends, I've never had the right words.

I have texted and said the words "I don't know what to say" more times than I can count. When I've fallen to my knees after hearing a test result from Kara. When I've watched her child play in the backyard while learning cancer had progressed to a new corner of her body and stolen yet another cell from her. What do you say besides "I don't know what to say" in these moments?

Our people aren't expecting us to solve anything or have perfect words. That's pressure we're putting on ourselves. The list of stupid things I've said to Kara is long and probably extends beyond what I even realize. In fact, some of those things have become the perfect opportunity to laugh when we want to cry.

I once asked Kara if it was killing her not to know something. That was an awful choice of words.

One friend jokingly referred to her own brain as weak, saying she needed to keep things simple, then realized what she'd said and that Kara had just finished brain radiation because of cancer growth. Kara had grace for her, and they ended up laughing about it.

Another time, Kara had just gotten out of the shower and had a towel wrapped around her head. A friend offered to brush Kara's hair, momentarily forgetting that Kara was bald at the time. Kara didn't burst into tears; she burst into laughter.

Upon learning Kara would lose her hair, another friend told her about the weird shape of her own skull and how she'd look funny if she were bald, quickly regretting her words.

While taking photos, a friend of Kara's mentioned she wanted to switch sides with her, that her hair was better on one side. (Amen, sister. Mine too.) A bald Kara turned to her and said, *"You don't need to apology-text me later about that comment. I know it's going to hit you and you'll feel bad."* Instead of being offended, Kara changed that into a moment they were able to laugh about.

We've done it all. We've said it all. Why am I sharing these stories? To show that you will say something you'll wish you hadn't. And you might even be able to laugh about it (after you bemoan what you said to a friend).

Through all this hardship, Kara has kept her sense of humor. One time when she wanted to know some news from me, she texted me saying she was dying to know.

The next text from her came in quickly: *"I'm actually dying, but I also want to know."*

How does a person answer that text? I think I laughed and then wanted to cry. Her ability to still see humor in the midst of horrible hard has been a blessing to all of us.

She's gone out of her way to make the rest of us comfortable, and she's taught us it's okay not to have perfect words. Kara reminds us that showing up matters, that community matters, even when we're simply there to listen and love.

Depending on the type of suffering a person is walking through, certain words can become land mines. Either we can allow them to explode into our lives and steal our joy, or we can answer with grace. Kara gives us such a gift when she is gentle with us. It's one of the reasons it's easy to be around her even when we say or do the wrong thing. She's not expecting perfection from us.

Are you the one walking a hard road? Do you have grace for those who are entering your life? What a huge difference it makes in forming beautiful friendships.

If I could be transported back in time to when my pastor was with us, I still wouldn't know what to say. But I would show up.

During this journey I have learned to be more comfortable with my uncomfortable. The more I've been around Kara, the easier it's become to not know what to say. I still struggle with it, but part of the ease has come from experience. From showing up without words. From showing up with the wrong words. From choosing to be there even when I don't know what to say or do.

I've also gotten braver with others who are suffering. I've started asking questions I wouldn't have asked before. Recently, while speaking to a person with a terminal illness, I asked her if she preferred to talk about her suffering or if she'd rather I didn't ask.

Communication is an amazing tool we can use to be gentle with one another.

I still can't believe I just asked her how she felt and what worked for her. This was a huge stretch for me. I am the queen of comfort. I don't like things that have even the potential for discomfort. I even like my clothes to be comfortable. When I walk in the door at night, the speed with which I change into pajamas is remarkable. The quest for comfort might even be my superhero power. So the last thing I'd ever want to do is make someone feel uncomfortable because I've brought up a subject they don't want to talk about or that I know is hurting them.

Because of that, in the past, I've played the let's-pretend-this-isn't-happening card.

But when a person is going through something hard and I don't mention *anything* about their trial, it's like a big elephant is sitting on my foot. I'm having to peer around the elephant to see and talk to them, but at no point do I mention the creature cutting off the circulation to one of my appendages.

Of course this scenario is silly, but not saying anything to someone about the suffering they are going through is a little like this.

Before this experience with Kara, I was so afraid to say the wrong thing that I wouldn't say anything at all. I was so fearful of hurting or offending that I didn't want to bring up the hard.

Please don't join me by overlooking the elephant on your foot.

Here's where the dance of walking through suffering with a loved one comes back again. Ignoring someone's suffering is hurtful. *Not saying anything at all is wounding.*

I've had many people reach out to me about Kara's story and comfort me, even just dropping a note to say they are praying for me. All the friends surrounding Kara have had this happen. We've been supported by the community around each of us. While it feels a little extravagant, considering that I'm not the one suffering, I covet those prayers. This isn't an easy road. But there are also people who say nothing to me, and that's awkward.

The same holds true for the person suffering. By not mentioning it, we're adding to the tension. My friend who lost her mother to cancer said that during the time her mom was sick, many people wouldn't say anything to her about her mom. They were so afraid to ask, so afraid to say the wrong thing, that they didn't say anything at all. She was going through something incredibly hard, and she remembers those moments as wounding.

We may feel feeble or inadequate, but making the point of saying *something* is better than saying nothing. While we aren't expected to have perfect words, phrases, and memorized Bible verses, we should at least express that we care.

Because we do care.

And when we don't say anything, it looks as though we don't.

None of us want that. We care so much that we go through the trouble of not bringing it up in the first place!

So, if we're supposed to say something, what should we say?

In the same way that it's okay to have a go-to meal, it's okay to have a go-to phrase. This doesn't cheapen your words or compassion. Tell that voice that says your words need to be spontaneous, not scripted, to shut up. Phrases like these work well:

I'm so sorry to hear about _____.

I'm sorry you're going through this. If you ever need to talk to someone, I'm happy to listen.

I'll be praying for you.

These are simple comfort phrases that express our sympathies for what someone is going through.

For those hungry for a definite in showing up for others, there is a guideline for helping us decipher what to say and what not to say when approaching suffering. An article in the *LA Times* titled "How Not to Say the Wrong Thing" provided a simple tool we can use.[1]

Their suggestion is to draw a circle with a number of rings around it. The name of the person who is suffering goes in the middle circle. From there, you can list others who are connected in various ways. The closer someone is to the one who is suffering, the closer their name goes to the center ring. And the key is this:

Comfort in, dump out.

---

1. Susan Silk and Barry Goldman, "How Not to Say the Wrong Thing," *Los Angeles Times*, April 7, 2013, http://articles.latimes.com/2013/apr/07/opinion/la-oe-0407 -silk-ring-theory-20130407. Illustration by Wes Bausmith.

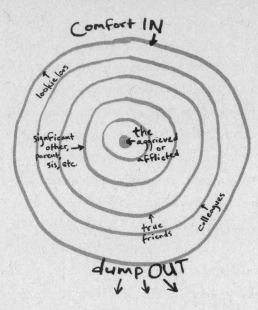

For example, I don't complain to Kara's family that she is dying. They are closer to the middle than I am. I don't tell them I thought Kara looked particularly sick one day or that her cancer is really hard on *me*.

That's not how it works.

But Jason could say those things to me. He can dump out to me about how he's struggling, because I'm on a ring that's farther out than he is. In the same way, I can turn to one of my friends who's outside of my Kara circle and lament that I'm losing my friend or that this is hard.

Use this as a general rule when dealing with suffering. Think of the person's proximity to the middle circle, and if they are closer in than you, use comfort phrases. No dumping in about what you're feeling. When you need to express your wounding and hurt, turn to people who are in a ring farther out than you are and express yourself there.

This seems logical, and I think many of us know instinctually that this is how it should be. But when we're caught off guard, we can easily say things without thinking.

The other morning I was talking to Jason in the school parking lot. He looked weary, and I was about to open my mouth and say how tough this is for all of us. But that statement would have included me. Because of this guideline, I changed my words and instead comforted in, which saved me from regretting that moment.

And if in doubt as to whether someone is closer to the middle circle than you, try to err on the side of comforting instead of dumping. Comfort is always received as a gift.

In an attempt to comfort, many Christians offer platitudes that point to Jesus. But phrases such as "God has a plan," "He won't give you more than you can handle," and "All things work together for good for those who love God" are not sympathetic. Platitudes like these are hurtful and wince-worthy.

When we learned Kara's cancer had progressed and would one day—barring a miracle—take her life, I spent many days crying at inopportune moments. People, in their efforts to comfort me, would tell me things like "God is still good," "He has a plan," and "Look at how God is using Kara to change lives."

These statements are completely true. I don't deny them. We can't even begin to count the number of people Kara has influenced. But did I want to hear this?

No.

At the time, I didn't know why they upset me so much. Later I figured out the answer: I already knew those truths. I knew God was still good, that He was going to be with Kara and her family and friends. I still believed. What I wanted in those moments was a hug. A nod of understanding. Someone to simply say, "I'm so sorry. This must be hard. I'll be praying for Kara and you."

Our people who are suffering know the truth of God's provision and grace. What they need is for us to express that we care and then to listen in love.

Let's give our people the room for this to be their story. We may have similarities in our stories, but this trial is unique to them. Saying something like "I know how you feel" or "I've been through something similar" makes it about us. Saying "I'm so sorry. I can't imagine how hard this is for you" keeps the focus on them.

We don't have to fill the silence with a bunch of words or tell the story of another friend who's going through a different trial. (I've done this. I'm totally wincing right now.) We don't have to barge in and ask hard questions in our attempt to say something.

Curiosity is different from caring.

These things have actually been said to Kara's friends or Jason:

"So, when is your wife going to die?"

"Is she close to the end?"

"Is she going to die soon?"

Curiosity wants to know what's going on. Caring wants the person to know they're not forgotten. Details aren't important.

I mentioned Christian platitudes, but does that mean we can't share a verse or an encouraging thought with our loved ones? Of course not. Our focus can and should remain on God—He is our hope in times of hardship, and we're all clinging to Him with a tight grip. But using biblical insight to try to explain the reasons behind someone's suffering isn't helpful. Share a Bible verse or bit of wisdom in order to encourage, not in an attempt to fix suffering.

If a verse or thought impresses you, share it by sending a note, card, email, or text. One friend who lives across town sent a note to Kara in the mail. It came on just the day she needed it, saying the words of encouragement she needed to hear.

When you're struggling for what to say, bite your tongue if you are tempted to suggest a miracle cure or offer phrases that "make everything all right." There are usually no explanations for the suffering that's happening to others. We live in a world where things don't make sense. There's hurt and hardship that we can't fix.

As for cures, the Internet bombards us with stories of people who "just did this" and long outlived their cancer or any predictions from doctors. Supposed cures for just about anything we can think of are at our fingertips. The desire to tap our fingers across the keys and seek out something to save our loved ones can be overwhelming.

We're problem solvers—fighters and scrappers. God made us this way for a reason. We've all had various things happen in our lives that have contributed to our strong natures. It's really not a surprise that so many of us want to help. But our desire to fix things can often get in the way of the silent support we can give by listening.

Right now, I'm watching an example of this unfold on Facebook. A woman has a granddaughter who needs special care and has a slew of high-risk doctors. The grandmother asked for prayers because the young girl is running a high fever. Instead of prayers—or at least along with prayers—she's being offered cures, questions, and advice:

"Have you done this?" "Take her to the ER!" "What about this?" This woman didn't ask for help or suggestions about what to do. She asked for prayers. So why are people bombarding her with advice instead of simply praying as she asked?

Most of the time our loved ones are not asking for solutions to their troubles. Often they just want someone to listen or to pray. Before giving advice or offering a cure, we should first consider whether the person asked for it.

A friend at church recently told me about a medical issue she was having. She then said, *"If you hear of anything or think of anything that might help, let me know."*

Permission to solve granted.

This is rare. Most of the time, people aren't asking. And yet we continue to ignore this very blatant sign that points to how we should be responding to them.

Remembering not to fix is a struggle for me and probably always will be. But I'm learning to listen and to fight the side of my nature that's only half listening because I've already started solving.

When Kara was first diagnosed, I, too, struggled with the fixing/curing temptation. I thought, *This is my friend and I love her, so if I hear of anything that might help, I should tell her.*

But this just isn't true.

Kara had a plan from the start with doctors she trusts. She knew what she believed in and what she wanted to do. And my job as a friend was to support her in that.

Thank goodness I had a wise person speak into my life as I struggled through what to say and what not to say. Her words were a lifeline. She said, *"This isn't your battle."*

I rolled those words around in my head for weeks, months even, coming to the conclusion that she was right. Kara's battle wasn't my battle. She was making decisions based on her own beliefs, fighting her cancer battle in the ways she chose to do it.

My job as a friend was to come alongside her in the decisions she made. We're like the support troops. We don't get to pull the trigger. We're running errands, making meals, helping where we can. But the health decisions come down to the person suffering.

If you're questioning whether you should say something to your person about a cure, please stop and pray for the Holy Spirit's guidance. And if at all possible, just don't say anything.

I've been the person to pick up a phone and call someone who was terminally ill, offering something I hoped would help. I know that tightening in my chest and the thought that what I had to say was utterly important.

I get it.

But I also regret making that phone call. Now that I've seen what it's like from the inside, I would err on the side of not saying anything.

One afternoon, Jason came home while Kara and I were hanging out. He walked in the room and mentioned what they'd been sent that day in terms of cures. The conversation seemed normal to them. I asked them how often this happened and they said all the time.

Sitting there with them, hearing those options, I felt overwhelmed. Something clicked in my head. From the outside, we are *one person* thinking of *one thing* that might help. But on the inside, numerous cures are being offered.

For the first time, I see the turmoil potential cures can create in the suffering person's world. Instead of bringing a ray of hope to the situation, the possible cure often distracts and overwhelms. In reality, those ideas may or may not work. If your person is suffering from an illness, know that you aren't the first person to offer them a cure.

Ask them if they want this kind of information, and if they say no, honor that.

What if you are certain what you have to offer your person is the difference between life and death? What if you've prayed and you still feel led to share something? What if you *absolutely cannot live with yourself* if you do not say something?

If you can't be deterred from sharing, consider carefully the approach you take.

Jason is a pastor, and he's often called upon to meet with people. Many times he doesn't know the subject they want to speak with him about until he arrives. When he was contacted by someone requesting a meeting, he went, not knowing exactly what to expect, but ready to serve in his pastoral role.

He thought the meeting was about how he could help this person.

When he arrived, the man blindsided him by giving him a folder containing details of a possible cure. Not only that, he wanted Jason to follow up with him. He wanted to know what Jason planned to do with the information.

Another man took a completely opposite approach. He was a trusted, wise person in Jason's life. He mentioned to Jason that he reads a lot and said that when he came across medical articles that might be of interest to Kara and Jason, he planned to forward them by email to Jason.

End of conversation.

Jason often ended up reading those emails and articles and even asking their doctors about them at times.

This man never checked in with Jason to find out what he did with the information he sent. By sending the articles in a nonintrusive way and then letting go, he made it about Jason, not himself.

Our desire to offer cures and fix things stems from a place of love, but there comes a point when we must trust in the sovereignty of God.

After I realized this wasn't my battle, I began to pray things like this: *God, please bring Kara to the doctor and treatment You have planned. If she's supposed to be doing a certain thing, will You direct her there? Give her and Jason wisdom as they deal with so many options, and make Your plan for them very clear.*

Jason and Kara have a trust in the sovereignty of God that is rare. They've prayed over their choices and asked for God's guidance. They believe that God is leading them and that, ultimately, Kara's life is in His hands.

Though we'd very much like to be in control, it's not up to us to save.

God's got us covered. I think our fear and panic come when we realize His answers might not be according to our desires. But the prayer we must pray is *Not my will, but Yours.*

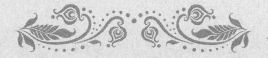

Kara

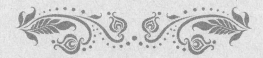

For those who know me, the title of this chapter ("The Gift of Silence") and my name in the same sentence is hilarious. I'm a talker. I think the sophisticated-sounding phrase is "a verbal communicator." But I've learned in this hard season that there are times when words are bitter, even if they may be true. You might think by reading Jill's words that honoring the silence was a challenge only for her. But it's been a challenge for me, too, to resist the urge to say something to try to make someone feel at ease. We've all had to grow in grace in this area.

People in the caring professions call this the "ministry of presence." It means what it sounds like, that you and I can perform a ministry by simply showing up and being there for someone. We don't have to say any special words. We don't have to have a lot of prayer experience under our belts. Our physical presence is enough. I believe God sometimes wants to say something to us in those situations but that His voice gets crowded out by our nervous talk, trying to say the right thing or come up with a comparable story. At times we need to be still and know that He is God and we are not.

But that's not to say words don't matter. There have been times when the presence of another person, coupled with Scripture being read, has been an amazing gift to me. My dear friend Carl has not missed an appointment, a procedure, a scan in almost two years. And he has been faithful to show up since I've been in hospice care. He comes by with his calming presence and prays and reads from the Psalms. Carl doesn't add any commentary or preach me a minisermon. He just reads the words. He's not trying to fix anything, but rather he's reminding me of things I know but may lose sight of when my vision is doubled and the pain is so intense. The time I spend each day with Carl has been like a sanctuary, a silence of words. I'm not sure if that makes sense or not. I know only how much it has meant to me.

1. Look back at the "Comfort In, Dump Out" illustration. Now consider the person you're showing up for and think about the people you can comfort. In the same way, think about the people you can "dump out" to. These groups won't change; in other words, you'll always be able to comfort a, b, or c, and you'll always need to dump to x, y, and z.

2. Okay, here's your chance. Write down two or three inappropriate Christian platitudes you've either heard said to others or been the recipient of yourself. There might be one you've even used before and after the fact thought, *Wow, that really wasn't helpful.* There's no need to feel shame. If anything, try to laugh about it. We all get do-overs in the practice of showing up.

Chapter 4

The Nurturing of Friendships

Today I simply want to scream. Kara says the answers from her doctor are as she expected, and if I'm allowed to be honest, they are for me too. I see her suffering, the way she doesn't feel well, and it makes my mind wander regarding what is happening, where the cancer is moving. But then there's the hope. The thing waving arms and saying things like, Maybe it will be gone. Can you imagine the miracle? Can you see the people rejoicing? But when it doesn't happen like that, where do I go? Usually tears. And then prayers. They aren't eloquent. They are usually short phrases, often one word. Jesus. Help. Do You see this suffering? But of course He does. He knows.

I love this friend of mine. I know so many who read her blog feel the same way. They've chosen to jump in with her, with her family, to care about someone they've never met. This I love. So often we see a blog post or someone else's suffering and we disconnect. I know I do. The suffering in this world can be too much.

Sometimes people tell me they can't read Kara's blog. They can't handle hearing about cancer. And that's *when I know they've never really read her blog. Because it's about life far more than it is about cancer. It's about kindness. It's about apologizing to my children when I lose my temper for the millionth time. It's about taking every moment captive. It's about stopping in the middle of an excellent chapter to be present with my children. She's taught me so much, and yet, she's just a friend. Just a mom who has kids in the same classes as my kids. Just a friend whose story isn't what she expected. Isn't what we expected. Just. Not. Some days it feels like nothing fits this story but a few words I might not otherwise think or say.*

Cristy remembers wanting to pursue a friendship with Kara during the first round of chemotherapy, but she felt caught between taking the step toward a deeper friendship and waiting for Kara to be done fighting cancer so that she could engage. Like many of us here, she knew that Kara already had great friends who were surrounding her in amazing ways. She didn't think Kara needed more people or had the energy for more friendships—certainly not while she was going through something so hard.

Cristy waited.

Now she looks back on that time and wonders what she was waiting for.

"Don't wait," she whispers. *"Don't wait for things to get better before pursuing a friendship, because things might not get better."* Once

she realized the cancer wasn't going anywhere, Cristy stopped waiting. Her friendship with Kara grew in the midst of Kara's cancer battle.

Many of us held back because we hadn't known Kara for very long before she got sick. We now realize this didn't need to keep us from growing friendships.

There's a lot of hard in our world. Just today, I've said I would pray for two friends regarding health issues and pray for another who was dealing with a troubled family relationship. Life is not easy. And if we wait for a time without hardship before engaging with others, we may never form relationships.

Whether you're entering someone's life before, during, or after suffering, it's never too late or too early to jump in.

Those who have read and followed Kara's journey have witnessed the way her family have been kept by their community. Many have asked themselves, *If I were to walk something hard, who would be there for me? Who are my people?* I've asked myself the same questions.

Kara preaches, teaches, and does big love, modeling community in a way that many of us haven't seen before. Countless people have been influenced by Kara's big-love approach to life and want to grow their community, but many don't know where to start.

I've learned from watching Kara that a house doesn't need to be perfectly clean and a meal eaten together doesn't have to be gourmet. People matter. Taking a step toward someone else matters. But for an introvert, this can feel like doing math. How do we even begin to do this? Isn't community something for those extroverts out there who want to talk to everyone?

My husband is an extrovert, and when we were first married and would plan a date night, he would inevitably ask me who we should invite to go with us. On a date.

In my young married-ness, I was often offended by this. I wanted to go on a date with just him. This was a foreign concept to him, not because he didn't love me or want to spend time with me, but because he's built for people. They energize him. Last night, my husband turned to me with amusement and told me his excitement about having three nights in a row with activities. This is something I often dread because while I might enjoy the events, they also zap my energy. We now laugh about our personality differences and this early miscommunication in our marriage.

Kara is outgoing like my husband. She refuels with people. When I see the way she draws people to community, I sometimes get so overwhelmed at the thought of doing the same that I want to forfeit the game before I've even started. It sounds like a lot of work to me, growing friendships. Perhaps I'd be better off reading a book and dealing with this at another time.

The good news for introverts like me, and maybe you, is that it's possible, and it's not even that painful. The tough-love news is that introverting is not an excuse for avoiding community—although I have attempted to use it as one before.

I'm definitely not perfect in this area. I still have days when hiding is easier, but I'm working on it. It's good to have someone you can use as a sounding board and who you can discuss your introvert tendencies with. I usually talk to my husband. He helps me decipher if I'm holing up, and he sometimes gives me a loving push to move me out of my introvert shell.

And if you are an extrovert, the title itself doesn't necessarily mean you're participating in community. Efforts must be made to build relationships, no matter what our Myers-Briggs test shows.

We need each other. God made us to walk with each other. Our style of community might look different than Kara's, but it still counts.

Some people love to cook and have guests over.

Others might get panicked by that thought.

Some are okay with welcoming people into a house that's well loved but not picked up.

Others want everything to be perfect before they open the door.

We're all made to be who we are for a reason, and we can find community within the parameters of our personalities.

The other night, we went to dinner with a couple to get to know them better. (Don't worry, this was planned. It wasn't a date my husband turned into a double date.) At first, I'd arranged to invite the couple over for dinner. But once we realized neither of us had kids that night, we switched to going out. By doing this, I was able to focus on getting to know them instead of concentrating on cooking or cleaning my house.

Kara is the queen of saying "Just come over," while I'm the queen of saying "Give me two days' notice."

Our versions of doing community look different, but that's okay. Unlike my friend, I am not the hostess-with-the-mostess type. The challenge is to begin where we are, where we are comfortable. Wait! Maybe one step beyond comfort. Because for some of us, if we stayed in the comfort zone, we'd never talk to a new person again.

Kara has challenged us over and over to let people into our houses and our lives even if they are messy. And who doesn't have a messy life? We might like to pretend we don't, but most of us do. Life isn't Pinterest, is it?

It's okay if you want to have someone over and you order pizza instead of cooking. It's also completely acceptable to go out to a restaurant. The point is to show up.

Start somewhere. Maybe with a cup of coffee while your baby crawls all over you and another mom nurses her infant.

If it's too much to pick up the phone, what about getting to know someone by text? (I know some of you are cheering right now. I, too, am all about texting, as I've already mentioned about fifty-six times.)

Some of us will need to start small. Even attempting to have a conversation with someone at school or work we might not normally speak to can be a huge first step.

Being introverted versus extroverted might change the landscapes of the friendships we develop. We might have fewer numbers, but there are still ways to grow community from our tentative perch.

If you're lonely and longing for friendship, you could even start to enter into community by serving someone else. We might think someone has all the friends they need when they are walking through hard, but that might not be true. Their help and resources could be limited. Your relationship might grow during another's suffering, like many of ours did.

My friend and I were recently discussing the season of being stay-at-home moms and the loneliness we felt during that time, especially with young kids at home and no kids in school yet. It can be a very isolating time. Designer heels, intense meetings, and work friends have been replaced with diapers, spit-up, and long days without much adult conversation.

I remember the loneliness of those days. I knew I needed community, but I didn't know where to start. Joining MOPS was my first step toward finding community during that new stage in my life.

Now I wonder when some of the people who currently surround me sneaked up on me. During those first steps, finding friendships was hard work. But then, bit by bit, it became easier. School became a huge community for me. I know the mothers there would support me if I needed them to, partly because I've seen them do it for Kara and partly because they already do take care of me and watch out for me in the smaller things in life.

Church has been another place that I've seen my community grow.

Even the girlfriends surrounding Kara have become a community for me. Each person Kara has in her life is unique and gifted, and my relationships with these women have grown out of this shared hardship.

In the midst of her suffering, Kara is a keeper and grower of friendships, a tender nurturer of those around her. I know she loves to garden, and I imagine her walking through rows of sprouts, pausing to check on each one as she does with her friends.

Many times Kara has asked me about other girlfriends, how they are holding up, if anyone has checked on them. She's always thinking about others. While going through something horribly hard, she still considers how much her cancer is affecting her friends.

Cultivating friendships before a hard season begins is something I've witnessed before. But watching someone continue to do the work of loving those around them even while they are suffering is not nearly as common.

This has been one of the most amazing things I've seen Kara do, and it's surprised me. Kara isn't selfish in her suffering. She's always conscious of others and works to not overburden her friends and family. Kara hasn't stopped loving and growing her community during her cancer. Things have changed, but she still works to open her world and to love big.

This is part of why Kara is so easy to love and show up for. She's not just taking. She really does give back to each of us in relationship with her. The look of that has changed as her cancer has progressed, but the roots that were planted early on continue to sustain our friendships when Kara isn't as able to engage with each of us as she once was.

When our two youngest were in preschool together, I would sometimes watch her daughter Story on days when the kids didn't have school. Having her over was great for both Kara and me. My kiddo got a playmate on a day off from school, and Kara had the help she needed.

The next year, my son had a different schedule from Story's. Kara never asked me to watch her daughter again because she knew I didn't have a kiddo at home for Story to play with. This always amazed me. She tries not to overburden her friends by asking the same people to always do the same things.

Kara found another family who filled the role beautifully—a mom who had a child the same age as Story. This mom took Story on the days she didn't have school.

Another friend who had a day off from teaching school offered to help Kara with something. Kara's reply? "No. That's your day off."

She's protective of her friends. Even when she's feeling awful, she's present in seeing what's going on in her friends' lives. She still uses her energy to invest in others. This is the way Kara honors her community. Yes, she might be suffering, but she still cares about her people.

During her second round of chemo, Kara continued to grow the community around her. She kept opening herself up to others at a time when most of us wouldn't have seen the reason for that or understood why we should continue to love so big.

While most illnesses or trials happen for a period of time and then end, Kara's was ongoing. She realized this could put a heavy burden on those closest to her. She didn't want to do that, and so she continued to build friendships even in her suffering. She pulled people into her life and grew the community around her so that we could support one another.

One night, in the middle of Kara's battle, a group of women gathered for a girls' night in. Kara had just received devastating test results showing cancer growth in her brain. She glanced at Shellie and me and said, *"You two would be perfect for each other."* Shellie and I didn't really know each other that well, and Kara was setting us up to be friends. We still laugh about it. (She nailed it, but we're totally not going to admit that to her.)

But for most of us, friendships won't be set up by a friend who has a terminal illness and is trying to take care of those around her. Relationships will take time and effort and then grow slowly.

If you question who would surround you during suffering but don't know the answer, now is the time to begin growing those friendships. They will bless you whether or not you end up walking through trials together. But in this world, the odds are that something tough will come at one of you. Facing the hardship together is so much better than facing it alone.

Kara

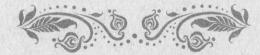

Facebook has almost single-handedly turned the word *friend* into a verb. I get it, but I don't really like it because *friend* is primarily a noun. In my life the word refers to a living, breathing person. Someone who has witnessed my body crumble under the weight of chemotherapy and cancer and stayed anyway. Someone who has hugged my children and provided meals for my family, who has listened to my heart and wept with me when we don't have answers to this hard. I have asked friends if my children are going to be okay when I'm gone, though I barely remember some of the conversations because medications steal my memory. I have told my friends I don't know how to die well, though I long to do exactly that. And they have met me there. Not always with answers—and I'm not sure I'm even looking for answers. But they've met me with friendship. I've chosen to make room in my life for them, just like they have for me. It's always a two-way street. And when I say "make room," I'm not using figurative language. I'm talking about literal room—in my house or at our dinner table or in my mind.

Nurturing friendships is hard enough when everyone is healthy. But when you show up and do the work of being a friend to someone who is suffering, it will cost you something. In other words, you're going to have to sacrifice your comfort, your schedule, and maybe even aspects of your faith.

That last phrase may have caught you off guard. It is a little strange to think about sacrificing pieces of your faith. But consider it for a minute. If you've never really walked with someone through suffering, and if your view of God up to this point has resembled a math equation (prayer + God = healing), then I'm sorry to have to tell you, but you're going to have to sacrifice pieces of that way of believing. If you can't, then forget about *nurturing* a friendship. And while giving up those pieces may hurt, it's not senseless pain. If you can stay soft and open to God during that time, you can begin to realize a bigger faith than you've had up to that point. I'm talking about growing up, becoming a woman or a man, and putting away the childish while keeping the childlike.

1. If you were asked to walk something hard, who would be there for you? Who are your people?

2. This one is not so much a question as it is a reminder. Walking with someone through suffering is going to stretch your faith. You may have to give up pieces of your faith, assumptions you may have grown up with or cultural ideas as to how faith is supposed to work. Remember, stay soft.

Chapter 5

The Art of Giving and Receiving

I had this thought, this vision of God coming in all His glory to end our suffering, and how Kara would be radiant because she believed. She'd be waving her hands saying, "Pick me up! Scoop me up! I'm ready. I never doubted You."

Where would I be? Somewhere to the side, a look of concern on my face. "I believed You a lot of the time. Especially when things were good."

I think there was a time I stopped believing.

It wasn't blatant. No one probably even realized it. I still went to church. I still talked about God and prayed. But something in me was quiet. Not on fire.

I knew Him, but I didn't believe Him. I believed in Him. But I didn't believe Him.

In a life that had been good, suddenly there was hard. And instead of believing God is good, I started to believe those whispers the world sends out. The ones that slither along your spine and quietly speak into your soul.

He must not love you, they say.

He can't. Not if He lets you endure this without rescuing you from it.

And even if the something is a small hard, those whispers gain momentum.

The questions start.

Only, when you're a Christian, you process the questions quietly. Because you know better. You know better. But those doubts begin to obscure everything else. Your faith stumbles. And you stop trusting Him one little piece at a time.

And then a friend comes along, and she's screaming, screaming in the midst of horrible hard that GOD IS STILL GOOD. That GOD IS SOVEREIGN. That SUFFERING IS NOT THE ABSENCE OF GOD'S GOODNESS.

And it's like a fire has started.

New whispers grow like unchecked flames.

What if those are lies? What if God is good in the midst of this? What if?

And then suddenly we begin to proclaim to the world: YOU HAVE LIED TO US, Satan, you deceiver. You tried to tell me suffering was the absence of God's goodness. But you are a liar and a snake.

And I don't believe you anymore.

I believe Him. I believe in His promises even when I don't understand them.

I believe. I believe. I believe.

Help my unbelief.

Kara has been asked to walk a very hard road—one might say the hardest here on earth—and yet she's accepted that. She has fought cancer's hold with everything in her, but she has also obeyed the Lord in accepting the path she's been asked to walk.

She's chosen to praise God and be grateful in the midst of hard.

This modeling of receiving is evident in many corners of her life, transferring to the way she's accepted help and support from those around her.

Accepting can come in many forms—the hard path God has asked us to walk, wisdom or advice from others, help meeting our physical needs.

All of these require humility, which is not innate to our natures. Well, perhaps it's in your nature, but not mine. If the thought of receiving makes you wince, welcome to the party. We can stand next to one another and commiserate on our lack of accepting skills. In the past, Kara would have been standing next to us. She probably would have been the party hostess. But over the course of her suffering, she's had to let go of doing everything herself.

She didn't have to accept help, but she chose to. And her journey and community would not be what they are today had she not made the decision to receive.

Shellie is a friend who went through the process of adopting a son. It was a long, long road, and she and her husband incurred many expenses while they waited years for him. She raised money for the adoption by saving, selling furniture she refinished, cleaning homes, and selling freezer meals. They even sold some of their possessions, willing to do whatever it took to get their son home. But the costs of adoption were still beyond what she and her husband could manage.

They had to ask for help. And even harder, they had to receive.

This is a quote from her blog during that time when her family walked their own unimaginable hard:

> I long for the day when all four of our children live under the same roof, when our life is dull again and we can be the givers instead of the receivers. It is so humbling to continually be on the receiving end of selfless love, encouragement, prayers, donations. I feel so unworthy. Sometimes I say to Jesus, "I'm humbled enough, right? Can I be done now?" I think the answer is no.

"I'm humbled enough, right? Can I be done now?" I love the authenticity in this because it truly is easier to give than to receive.

But in the same way that Kara's community has been shaped by her graceful receiving, Shellie's has too. The people who surrounded her during the time of painfully waiting for her son to come home are now invested in her family and in him. That community wouldn't exist had there not been a need and acceptance of others meeting that need.

Receiving is hard work. But what gracious receivers these friends have become.

Recently a friend offered to bring us a meal. I'd spent the night in the hospital with Kara, and I was weary. I thanked my friend but refused her help. I didn't know how to accept it. All I could think was that I wasn't the one suffering. Getting little sleep for a night was nothing compared to Kara's battle. I had no reason to complain, no reason to accept help.

I went to work that day, then headed home for an evening of getting the kids fed and ready for bed. We had no food prepared, and I ended up having to purchase something. I thought of my friend's offer and knew I should have accepted it. She's from a different circle than my Kara circle, and she wanted to show up for me while I was showing up for someone else. But I didn't let her, while Kara did let me. I wasn't playing fair.

It didn't matter that I didn't feel worthy of my friend's help or that my need wasn't as great as Kara's. What matters is that giving and receiving are building blocks of community, and I refused to let that happen.

Before getting sick, Kara loved being the one leading young women, mentoring and asking the questions. But when life threw unexpected things her way, the teacher had to become the student too. She realized the way to stay in community was to let others help her.

She is willing to let us in, even into the things she wants to cling to. Children's clothes being sorted. Meals cooked. Laundry folded and most likely put away in the wrong drawers. She lets us in. Can you imagine, as a mom, giving up so many of those things that make you feel like a mother?

When a friend's mother was battling terminal breast cancer a few years ago, there was a stretch of time when her mom was in hospice care and the family wanted to be with her daily. They had to accept all sorts of help. My friend said she struggled at first with accepting, especially since a lot of the help came from outside of her group of friends and from her parents' circles instead.

Her mother spoke into her struggle: *"People need to help, and we need to let them. It's part of their processing."* My friend came to the conclusion that letting people help was just as important as their offering to help.

How beautiful that even in her suffering, this wise woman saw that accepting help was a way to love those around her.

From the outside, there's not a lot we can do for our loved ones in terms of making things better. We can pray. We can't make an illness go away or fix their troubles. So when we have the opportunity to help our loved ones, we want to do things well. We want to make it as easy as possible for those suffering to accept our help.

I mentioned this earlier in the book, but it bears repeating because this theme was mentioned over and over as I spoke to people about suffering: when offering to help, be specific. In grief and suffering, people don't have the capacity to make decisions as they normally would. The more detailed we can be, the better.

"Can I pick up your kids on this day, at this time, and take them here?"

Even if I wasn't going through something hard, I'd say yes to that offer.

With that much detail, they can answer yes easily or tweak the option you've given them.

People aren't ignoring us when we offer to help in blanket ways. They aren't trying to offend or not accept help. It's just that most of the time, they don't know how to answer.

One friend who was going through something hard explained it this way:

> When someone says "Just let me know what you
> need, okay?" how am I supposed to respond?

Should I say that I need someone to mow my lawn and I haven't cleaned my house or done laundry in weeks? Of course not. What if they feel uncomfortable with what I need? I don't want to intrude in someone's life like that. But if someone said to me, "I'd like to come over, run the vacuum through your house, and throw in a load of laundry," now that's different. If they offered something concrete like that and insisted on showing up, it would be far easier to accept their help.

Offering specifics not only gives us the opportunity to serve in an area we're gifted in but also allows people to begin to accept help more easily.

In our sphere with Kara, there's been a balance of giving and receiving. Efforts have been made on both sides to do our part well. Certain things have worked well for us, and they can easily be transferred to your own story of showing up.

One big way Kara has given back to us is by keeping us informed of what's going on. She's blogged and been very open during her whole journey. During Kara's chemotherapy treatments, people would often ask me how she was doing, and I wouldn't know more than what she'd said on her blog. She was great about keeping us updated in that way.

While I completely understand the need to keep certain things private in suffering, figuring out what you're willing to share and then finding an avenue to do that is a big blessing to those around you. It helps them know how to pray and how to help, in addition to giving them a way to know how you are and what's going on without having to ask.

Keeping your people informed—however you decide to do that—is one of the best gifts you can give back. Hopefully this sharing will also prevent people from pestering you about what's going on. You could even state it this way: "I'll be sharing updates here [list your preferred method], and I'd appreciate not being asked for details beyond that."

Communicating makes the process of showing up easier for both sides.

We currently text Jason before we go visit Kara. He's become the gatekeeper—and we appreciate his role in this. We want to be told no if Kara is having a tough day and can't have visitors. We trust him to tell us the truth about whether we should come.

I know I mentioned earlier my lack of skills in taking meals to friends in need, but this is, of course, an amazing hands-on way to help a suffering family and take a daily task off their list.

One way the Tippetts family have made this easier for all of us is to put a cooler on their front step. Meals can be dropped off in the cooler any time of the day, and those leaving them don't need to worry they might wake Kara or disrupt family time. It's a simple tool that's made taking a meal to them so much easier.

A suffering household can't deal with the logistics of returning dishes, so a way to love our people is to take dinner in disposable dishes or ones that don't need to be returned. That sounds so simple, but it's often overlooked.

If the suffering family can give out a list of meals they like and include a list of dislikes, this is also extremely helpful. The more guidelines and input from the family, the easier it is to surround them. Details matter, and this will help provide the kinds of meals the family will actually eat.

Remember, these families—these kids—are missing their mom's (or dad's) cooking. It's not going to be an easy road. The meal you made with so much love won't be perfect to their little mouths because it's not made by the right hands. This has nothing to do with you. So if they don't like your meal or don't consume every ounce of it, remember hearts are hurting during suffering and any lack of enthusiasm for a meal isn't about you.

At the front door to the Tippetts family's house, there's a chalkboard sign that gives instructions or updates: *Please don't ring the bell; immune suppressed; use hand sanitizer* (of which they have a big jug available for use). It's a way for them to communicate easily with people entering their home, and it prevents them from having to repeat themselves. Hopefully it's also a reminder for people who are sick not to enter but to come back when they are healthy.

Grocery shopping is another area we can step in and help. During Kara's first round of chemotherapy, she had two volunteer lists going—one for making meals and one for grocery shopping. Kara covered the cost of the groceries but needed someone to physically do the shopping. The family can make a specific list to be filled each week or can give general ideas of what they need.

If there are kids in the family, including items easily packed in lunches is another way to help. Packing lunches for four kids was an area that made Jason feel overwhelmed. Kara informed friends of this, and many stepped in and quietly took care of this task.

Recently, the teachers at school have taken it upon themselves to pack lunches for the children, completely shouldering this load for Jason and Kara. This is another tangible way to help. Something simple you can do from your home, such as packing one extra lunch for someone in your child's class, can feel like the greatest gift to another family. Plus, the kids feel big love in those amazingly well-packed lunches.

Going to the doctor can be overwhelming, and friends with medical backgrounds can be a big help. Offering to go along to listen and take notes with a loved one can be an amazing gift. Later, you'll be able to help them remember what was said and clarify things they may have missed.

Another practical way to help a suffering family is to appoint one person to be the contact for various needs. This way the family has one person to contact, who can then inform the troops of what's needed, and in turn those helping on the outside can go to this person with questions and offers instead of overwhelming the family.

In terms of the kids, you can help in several ways. For example, you can arrange playdates; provide transportation to and from school, birthday parties, and other activities; and assist with homework. Homework can be especially hard for a family that's going through suffering. A project that's time consuming for a typical family can sink a family struggling to keep their heads above water. Numerous parents have come alongside Jason and Kara's kiddos for tough school projects. They've sat with them and guided them through sometimes hours of homework, helping the children complete projects that needed to be done.

At our house, keeping kids in right-sized clothing can feel like a full-time job. This is another area that can be a way to give. If you have like-aged kiddos, include your friend's child when you take your own child shopping for necessary items. This can be a fun experience—they get to shop with a friend, and it's a way to provide an outlet for them should they need to talk with someone about the hard their family is going through.

Another gift that's a blessing to the family is photographs. Jen is a friend of Kara's who has taken photos of the Tippetts family along the whole journey, capturing so many priceless images. If you are a photographer, this is a gift you can offer. If not, donating a photo package to the family is an amazing way to show up for them.

People have also offered to sort mail, bills, cards, and gifts that come through the door. This is another area that can feel overwhelming to a suffering person. Helping decipher and sort medical bills, and then making sure they are being paid correctly by the insurance company, is another job that can reduce stress.

Depending on how ill a person is, offering to sit quietly at the house with them allows the rest of the family to do something outside of the home without feeling as though they are leaving their person alone.

One of the great ways Kara has met us in our giving is being willing not only to receive but also to ask. Her bedspread recently needed to be mended, and she asked a friend to come make a few stitches. This friend mentioned that had Kara not asked, she would never have known it needed to be done. Not only was she happy to do it, but she also got to visit with Kara in the process.

There is a group of women I often contact before I approach Jason and Kara. We've all started going to one another with questions, concerns, and attempts to figure out what the Tippetts family needs. We're usually able to solve issues of meeting needs without overwhelming the family with our questions. We're not professional caregivers or anything like that; in other words, you could form a group just like ours. If the group ever becomes a place to gossip, then it needs to be disbanded. This is a place of support, another tool for taking pressure off the family, not a place for speaking dishonoring words in any way. Set this ground rule at the outset and it will help keep the culture positive.

The people who have surrounded Kara amaze me. So many little things are quietly taken care of, and each person has their own way of showing up for Kara. People have given massages, cleaned her house, dropped off chopped firewood, painted her toenails, organized the garage. The list is pretty much endless, which proves that whatever is on your heart to do is likely exactly where you should begin.

Please, throw guilt, duty, and checklists aside. Our people know when our giving comes from a happy, loving heart versus a guilty heart. If I were walking through hard and knew someone had offered to help me out of a sense of duty, I wouldn't want that help. Our suffering friends don't want those attempts from us. They don't bless either party in the same way.

So, if God is calling us to show up for one another, is it ever okay to say no? Are we allowed to have boundaries? Or should we throw ourselves on the altar of serving one another?

With the sense of desperation we feel about Kara's illness, it can be tempting to go to the point of exhaustion wanting to help. But this isn't healthy. And overdoing in the area of showing up isn't what we're promoting. Part of the reason Kara's community has functioned so well is because so many have stepped up and done their part. We all have our own lives and responsibilities to take care of and families to be present with. There should be no guilt in taking care of the life God's given you.

My mom is often the person who listens to me as I process what Kara is going through and my feelings regarding her suffering. She lets me vent but then gently prompts me to go home and take care of my family—to not forget them in my desire to help Kara.

When Kara first found out about her cancer diagnosis and knew she needed six months of tough chemo, Heather felt the prompting of the Holy Spirit to show up for her. This friend committed to spending one day a week at Kara's house, doing whatever needed to be done and bringing a playmate for Kara's youngest. At that time, she and Kara didn't know each other in the way they do now, so stepping into this role was a stretch for Heather. She didn't have a clue what her showing up would look like, and it even changed from week to week. But when she felt the tug, she listened. Heather and her husband decided she would say no to some other things in her life during that period so that she could protect the energy and time she needed to devote to her own family as well. Having a boundary protected her from saying yes out of guilt to things that would have drained her and affected her family negatively.

Justine is the mom who's beautifully caring for the Tippetts kids right now, and she's made a decision to bypass some of the other things she would normally help with in order to keep filling the role at this time. This is a wise decision, considering all the emotions that come with caring for the children.

Boundaries are healthy for those of us on the outside, as well as for the family suffering. They protect us so that we'll be able to keep showing up for each other, and they are an important piece of giving and receiving well.

Kara

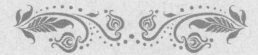

Jason and I originally thought we were coming to Colorado Springs to lend our strength to a group of people planting a church. We had no idea we were coming to offer our weakness. But that's what God had in mind. I'd like to say we had to learn the art of receiving, and we did, no doubt. But the longer we've walked through this season of suffering, we've seen that those two words—*giving* and *receiving*—get blurred in Jesus. We have received so much from others, but I believe if you were to ask them, they'd say they've been on the receiving end. It's funny, isn't it? When weakness and vulnerability are the foundation, it seems like everybody wins.

Jill's right. It is so much easier to give than to receive. It's just plain hard to receive, and even harder to ask. But there have been so many times when I've seen people suffer needlessly because they refused to ask. This wasn't because they weren't able to, like they were in a coma or something like that. It was because they were stubborn. I had that stubborn edge to me, too, before cancer came along. You can call it being independent, if you want, but it's just a few inches away from stubborn. Throughout this whole ordeal, Jason has encouraged me to have a soft heart—soft enough to give, to receive, and even to ask. That's what Jesus wants from us too, dear friend. He wants us to stay soft, to stay open to His goodness in a world in which there are so many days that can make us hard and bitter. Jesus wants us to give and receive. And, yes, He wants us to ask as well.

1. Recall the last time you received help. Was it hard to receive? Why or why not? Did you have to ask for that help? If you had to ask, how did that feel? Is that something you are used to doing or was that out of the ordinary for you?

2. Think about the other people who are showing up in the life of your loved one or friend who is suffering. Are you in contact with them in any way? Are you coordinating your care efforts, or are you showing up solo? The ladies who have surrounded Kara may sound extraordinary, but they're not. What they have been is willing, and God has blessed that willingness.

Chapter 6

The Battle of Insecurity

My jaw aches. It started sometime this afternoon. I took my kids to the pool, dreamed and brainstormed for a book living in my head, and yet still, this ache remains. I know it's from stress, but I'm not stressed. Nothing to be upset about here. It's a beautiful summer day. I'm not on a deadline. My kids run through the pool like wild children, passing other children in their wake. I am so thankful for their strength, for their endless energy, for their bodies. What a joy to watch them, what a blessing to have these moments. What is wrong? I ask my body, but it doesn't answer. We go home, have dinner. Still, I feel the tension, but I don't know what's wrong with me. I sit on the couch and tell my husband about my jaw aching. "What do you think it is?" I ask him. He says one word: "Kara."

My eyes instantly fill with tears. Yes. A breath shudders out of me. Of course. Of course. I've prayed for her today, for the Tippetts family. They are taking a trip, going to a dude ranch. And I've thought about what she's thinking about. She's dying. Typing the words, saying the words, makes me want to ... I don't know. Sometimes I think I'm going to be sick. Other times, I want to yell. Today, I cry.

Yes, that's what I'm upset about. I've been thinking about this vacation, about what Kara will be thinking about, and I know she'll be wondering if it's her last. She'll be squeezing out every moment. And while the rest of us squeeze out vacation moments with joy, Kara's joy will be mixed with desperation. She's choosing grace, she's choosing Jesus, but still, that knowledge is always there. I don't know for sure what she's thinking. I only know what I would do, what I would feel like. I would never function as well as Kara. But I know she's struggling. I read the posts about what pulled her out of bed, and I know what she's not saying, what she's protecting her children from. Oh, Jesus. Where are You in this?

You're there. Jason mentions the peace that shouldn't be, and I know it's You, God.

Will my jaw ache go away? Maybe. Probably not. Because my friend is ill. And there's nothing I can do. Nothing but pray and trust. And for a problem solver, that's a tough place to be.

⟨⤙⟩

Cancer and suffering are going on, and yet we keep having all these feelings. All these human feelings. Hurt. Jealousy. Insecurity. It seems when a friend is going through hard, these emotions should just stop. Our hearts should obey logic and not get jealous or feel insecure. These pesky feelings should pause because more important things are happening.

How can we be thinking about ourselves when our loved one is suffering?

Because we're human. And sinners. And knowing better doesn't make the doubt go away. Knowing not to be upset doesn't make our gut stop churning.

If anything, the emotions while walking through hard with a loved one are even more heightened than usual. We care deeply. We hurt intensely. We feel left out and sad or included and amazing. Far away. Nearby. No one is immune to the virus of insecurity.

When searching through my old writings for something to fit at the beginning of this chapter, I couldn't find a piece that felt "just right." I finally left a note for my editor stating that, to which he replied that what I had was "just fine." Oh, the irony of being insecure about my opening for the chapter about insecurity!

Early on in Kara's journey, a group of girlfriends planned a time to pray for Kara. I didn't learn about it until the photos were posted on Facebook. Those pictures surprised me because what followed was a hurt I didn't want to admit. And even though I knew better—I knew it was an oversight that I wasn't invited—I had a hard time shaking that feeling. It took me a few days to get over it.

Opening up Facebook and seeing something we weren't invited to is tough stuff on a normal day. But during a time when a friend is suffering and doesn't have a lot of energy to give to others, those photos, those doubts, can take you out at the knees.

At one point during my friendship with Kara, I went into a real tailspin of insecurity. (A separate time than the prayer meeting incident. Yes, I've done this more than once.) Whispers ate at me, telling me that my friend wasn't really my friend, that I wasn't important to her.

And I sank into those lies.

Insecurity had me doubting and thinking about myself and *my* issues for weeks on end. And then, because I was embarrassed to even be thinking what I was thinking while my friend was sick, I buried those feelings.

But they didn't go away. They ate at me.

I talked to my husband about it. *"Kara is sick. Why am I thinking about myself? It shouldn't be about me!"*

I prayed about it. *God, these thoughts are outrageous. Please make them stop! I don't want to think like this.*

But knowing my insecurities were wrong didn't stop them from happening. Insecurity is a backstabbing jerk that demands attention and doesn't listen to logic.

Weeks went by. I prayed. I asked God to take away the doubts and feelings. I kept fighting them because I knew in my heart they were wrong. *I knew it.*

But still, they gripped me.

Until one day, I finally came up with a plan. Every time I doubted or felt left out or questioned my relationship with Kara, I prayed *for her.* I didn't ask for the strange feelings to be removed from me anymore. I changed tactics and began to pray for her. For her family.

The insecurities, for me, were instantly gone. Snap your fingers, Superman-fast gone.

Just like that.

Satan won that battle for weeks because I let it be about me. About how I felt. And by simply changing my focus to praying for my friend, everything shifted.

I didn't tell Kara about my insecurities until after I'd worked through them. When she heard, she gently reassured me things were fine between us.

And then she told me I wasn't the only one feeling that way. Others had had the same experience. Our ages or what place we filled in her life didn't matter—many of us struggled with insecurities.

Another friend, hours away and in a completely different story as far as her relationship with Kara is concerned, found the same results I did through the same avenue. But as soon as she realized what was going on, she dropped what she was doing and began to pray for Kara. What took me weeks to figure out took her only minutes. Thank goodness some of us are wiser than others.

One particular story I love is about a girlfriend who served and showed up for Kara in countless ways. She wanted a deeper friendship with Kara, but she feared it would never develop. She was serving where God asked her to, but she also craved time and relationship. She began to feel upset about this, but she didn't say anything to Kara.

Many of us friends have done this along the way when we're upset about something, not because we think Kara doesn't care, but because there's a sense that we know better than to burden her with our doubts. She's sick, yet we're the ones needing reassurances.

So instead of bogging Kara down with these concerns, our sweet friend went to the Lord with her petitions. She prayed about wanting more friendship with Kara, and as is often the case, the answer she received was not the one she wanted. She was supposed to give Kara up—give up that desire to deepen their friendship—and hand that control over to God.

Though it wasn't easy, she obeyed. She opened her hands and said, *Not my will, but Yours.* You'll never believe what happened next. Okay, maybe you will, since you probably know the wonders of our great God.

He gave this friend a cherished and special friendship with Kara.

She glows when she talks about this story. What a victory that was for her in Christ. To give Kara up and then to have that friendship gifted back was amazing. She did what God asked of her, and He gave her the desires of her heart.

When we bring the focus back to God, He once again makes this journey about Him and not us, and we're blessed in the process.

Insecurity has been a theme for many of Kara's friends. And why wouldn't it be? Lives are changing because of Kara. She's touching so many people. When Satan is losing one battle, he's smart enough to switch tactics to another. And insecurity is the easiest way for him to get us to focus on ourselves under the misguided notion that we're thinking about the person suffering.

When Kara and I spoke of my insecurities, she told me something she's told each person surrounding her: *"You can trust me. You can trust in our friendship. There's nothing wrong between us, and if there is, I'll come to you about it."*

I don't think I've ever had another woman say this to me. What freedom Kara gives us in this statement.

She's often said that cancer doesn't give her the time to do drama and that she wants her friends to trust that she would come to them if there was an issue to be discussed.

What a breath of fresh air.

Even as I'm writing these words, they are a balm to my soul. Cancer steals so much from us, and our relationships aren't the same now as they once were. I miss Kara already, and she's still here. Many friends have also uttered these words.

We miss her. We miss what we once had.

So this reminder that she loves us, that it's not a fickle love, is such sweet grace. Cancer might hoard time, but the roots of those relationships are still the same and are untainted by this monster.

One friend put it this way:

> I have definitely struggled with insecurity, but I think Kara is so good at being straightforward and articulate that I feel like I can utterly trust her and her love. So during the stretches I don't hear from her for a while, while my tendency might be to feel insecure or wonder if I have hurt her, I don't have to fear because I know she would tell me if she were upset or if she needed something. When I have felt insecure in how to reach out to her and love her, I just press in toward her, again trusting her to be open and honest with me.

This is exactly what Kara wants from us, and many of us have pressed in toward her at times when we felt we didn't know what we were doing. She has asked us to trust her and our friendship with her, and so that's what we've worked to do.

One time, Kara and I were texting after disappointing test results. She told me not to come over, and I listened. I trusted her to tell me the truth, but I had a very uneasy feeling. Something about it didn't settle right, didn't fit with Kara's normal choices.

When I saw her and questioned her about it, she admitted she'd been hiding away from the world. I felt crushed that I hadn't followed my instinct and gone over regardless of what she said. But because Kara is always so honest with us about how she's feeling, I had no way of knowing she was hiding.

I told her, *"Next time, I'm just showing up. No more pushing away."* She agreed that she would be honest about her feelings in the future as she'd always been in the past.

Some people are this way, saying one thing and meaning another, but Kara typically is not that way. She's very open. But she's also human. So we worked through it.

Perhaps your friend is one who says not to come but who really wants you to just show up anyway. You're going to have to delve into the personality of your loved one and have some honest conversations about what showing up looks like between you.

This can help with the moments of insecurity.

There will also be times when you'll have to differentiate between your friend hurting you and their suffering hurting you. If something wounds you while you're walking through suffering with a loved one, ask yourself this: *Is my friend disappointing me? Or is this their illness or hard season disappointing me?*

Many times you'll find it's the latter.

But even if we realize it's the suffering disappointing us, not the person themselves, it can still hurt. A wound is a wound, no matter how it comes about.

It's okay to admit the hard a friend is going through is also stealing from us. It's okay to admit hurt. Just don't confess it to your suffering friend. Remember, comfort in, dump out.

Does this mean you can never talk to your friend about your own hard? Of course not. If you're going through suffering of your own, it's okay to talk about this with your loved one. Kara always says she's not trying to win at having the hardest hard. We all have trials, and it's okay to have a tough day. We don't have to keep silent about our own lives.

In these last few weeks as Kara's gotten sicker and her body isn't doing what she wants it to, her texting responses have gotten slower and are even nonexistent at times. She knows it's happening and mentioned it the other day when a few of us girls were visiting. It would be easy to let insecurity flare up again and wonder why she doesn't respond. But this is just another way that cancer is disappointing us. Kara doesn't want to be dying and losing pieces of herself. She doesn't want to miss out on her family and friendships. She doesn't want to be unable to respond to texts. She doesn't want the changes either, but they roll in without regard to how any of us feel.

Yesterday's Kara wouldn't leave a text without responding to it. But today's Kara doesn't have the strength to respond to all the messages coming her way. As friends, we have to work to differentiate between our friend hurting us and the circumstances hurting us.

This is a tough road, and navigating friendships in it even more so.

During suffering, relationships will change without your permission. And when a loved one is no longer capable of the relationship you once had, there will be mourning and a fight for a new normal.

With Kara in hospice care, our friendships have shifted once again. We're all struggling to find our footing. Now we text Jason before we go over. We are careful not to be too taxing on Kara, and yet, at times, we just feel so needy to see her. We need each other, whether it's just to sit together in silence or to grab a precious moment of friendship.

When I think about losing Kara, I get panicked. Does she know how we feel about her? Does she know we love her?

Of course she knows. In my more logical moments, I rest in this knowledge. I realize nothing we can say or do will make this process any easier. I used to think there was a way to prepare for letting go of her. But now I'm not sure there's anything we can do beforehand to prepare for after.

Are there enough words to fix this? No. We, as friends, have to rest in the knowledge that she knows our love, that we have hers, and that God will handle the rest.

Blythe, a friend who has walked closely with Kara, put these feelings so perfectly into words:

> I've experienced walking through suffering with
> people who seem altered or who can't do friendship
> as they once did, but it's always been temporary.
> Once they're better or have learned to do life in
> grief, etc., our relationship is restored. But with
> Kara that won't happen until heaven. So I think, do

I despair? I try to remember the reality of heaven and our relationship not only being restored but being better and more laugh filled and intimate and deeper than ever!

Barring a miracle, we aren't going to have a reconciliation on this earth of our friendship with Kara. We're not going to move beyond these pieces into wholeness again until heaven.

Whatever your person is struggling with—depression, illness, a disorder, a life event—the relationship you once had on this earth may or may not come back to you.

If restoration doesn't happen here, we do have the hope of it in heaven. There, the beauty of our relationships will be multiplied so many times over.

There will be times as we're fighting insecurities that it will be necessary to gain wisdom and insight from another person. As long as this avenue is pursued in an *I'm struggling* way instead of an *I'm gossiping* way, friends can be a huge help in processing our insecurities and speaking the truth we're having trouble hearing.

In Kara's situation, her energy is precious. I don't want to waste it on dissecting something I'm struggling with. Sometimes a word of truth from a friend is enough to calm my doubts and concerns.

Walking through hard with loved ones is a new world, and having help navigating it is such a blessing. Kara always says, "I've never done this before. Have you?" And we say no. Because we're really all stumbling through this together.

As we've entered the hospice stage, Kara's circles have gotten smaller. She has always been such a gatherer of people, such a master at community, that not having the energy to pursue all her friend-ships is hard for her and for those around her.

I want to reach out and hug the people who are feeling the loss of friendship with Kara. I want to whisper to each person, "You still matter."

When relationships change because of hardship, please don't discount what you had. It's not because of something you did or didn't do. It's simply the nature of suffering. It takes things that were previously beautiful and tries to taint them.

Don't let it. Those moments, those friendships, all matter. Even if they don't look the same as they once did.

Insecurity is not your friend, but it's going to try to be. It's going to attempt to consume your thoughts, to tell you that you're not important and you should back away. It's going to tell you that your relationship is one-sided.

At times those thoughts may feel more like the truth than anything else. But insecurity is a liar. Lean into God and let your insecurities be covered by His truth. Look through His filter. Fight these feelings by praying for the other person and putting your focus back on God and others.

And if you have to do this on repeat for it to work for you, that's okay. Once again, we can stand next to each other at the party.

Kara

His was a gentleness of necessity. Not what He should or ought to do. But what He must. He lived as a man might live only near the end of his life, in a way that militates against putting off what one has to do.

I have a friend who wrote those lines about Jesus. Even though I often fail, that's how I've tried to live as a wife and mother and friend dying of cancer—with *a gentleness of necessity*. It's kept the drama to a minimum. I'd love to tell you it's done away with the drama entirely, but I'd be lying. There's always a little drama. But the big dramas? I just don't have time for them. I hope you smiled at that sentence, because I did. Being gentle doesn't mean taking it easy on somebody. It actually means being very brave—brave enough to be honest and direct and do or say what you must do or say.

I'm not sure if men battle insecurity like women do. My gut tells me they do, but they'll never admit it. A big part of showing up is admitting that we feel insecure about this or that. We may confess that to a friend, or it might be a conversation we have with ourselves. The main thing is that we don't try to hide those feelings but instead shine a light on them. I'm convinced this is a daily practice.

Confess yours sins to each other and pray for
each other so that you may be healed.

James 5:16

We usually think about sins as the biggies—murder, theft, adultery, and so on. But if *sin* means "missing the mark," then I'm pretty sure insecurity is fair game. Insecurity keeps you and me from living the kind of life God desires for us. We miss the mark. So confess to a friend or your spouse. You may find he or she is insecure too. Pray for each other, and then pay attention to the many ways God's healing shows up in your lives.

1. There are annoyances in our lives, small things that can frustrate us. Then there are battles, things that take all our courage to face. Insecurity is in the battle category. It is one of the tactics the Enemy uses to cause us to doubt ourselves. When was the last time you felt insecure, and what was going on during that time? How did you handle it, or did it handle you?

2. The most effective battle plan is to cover yourself with God's truth. You can be insecure, or you can be secure in Him. Do you have a go-to prayer or verse you use to combat insecurity? Here are a few verses that we've used. You may have others that are particularly powerful for you. Don't hesitate to read them, speak them, pray them—whatever you have to do to keep God's truth in front of you in the battle.

- 1 John 4:4—"You, dear children, are from God and have overcome them, because the one who is in you is greater than the one who is in the world."
- John 14:27—"Peace I leave with you; my peace I give you. I do not give to you as the world gives. Do not let your hearts be troubled and do not be afraid."
- 2 Timothy 1:7—"For the Spirit God gave us does not make us timid, but gives us power, love and self-discipline."

Chapter 7

The Highs and Lows Together

Today was one of the good days. Kara has been pretty much bedridden for weeks, and suddenly, a new medicine, and she's herself. She's herself with a leg full of cancer, but she's puttering around her house, cleaning and putting things away.

I haven't seen her putter for months.

I can tell she feels so great today. Pain and tiredness have lifted and been replaced by a covering of medicine. Medicine that's working. It's glorious.

It's scary.

I always tell people I've said stupid things on this journey, and today I did exactly that.

Kara was putting dishes in the dishwasher and I said I wanted her to stop. I wanted her to sit down. To not overdo. Stupid? Yes. But that's where my heart was. I wanted to protect her.

Jason and Mickey were there, and they just smiled and nodded their heads—though they know better than to say something. They might agree with what I feel, but they are kind enough to know Kara needs these moments after being locked in a bed for so long.

None of us want a day tomorrow when Kara will have to deal with the pain that overdoing today caused. Yet I'm the one who opened my mouth and said it.

I already know my comment is forgotten . . . at least I hope. But for me, it will go to the graveyard that holds all the things that didn't need to be said.

While I'm chiding myself for being . . . myself, I'm also praising Jesus for how Kara feels. So many have been praying for a miracle. What if we're witnessing it today? To see Kara up and around is breathtaking. When all these pieces of her are being ripped from our hands, something is given back to us. She's ours for today. Today is one of the good days after many, many days of lows. We'll take it. We'll rejoice in it. And if the pain comes tomorrow as I fear but hope not, then we'll have the memory of today as the beautiful gift it was. But I am going to pray this good day repeats itself. There are moments to be claimed yet.

Story has a mother's tea at school in a week, and Kara wants to go. She's praying it will be one of the good days so that she can attend.

There was even talk of the beach today.

So I will pray over those moments.

And I will hold on to today. Thank You, God, for one of the good days.

I will try not to be greedy. I will try not to think of the moments to come or fear the days without her.

I will try to live in today.

❧

I don't know how to do this is a thought that has entered my mind more times than I can count while walking through hard with Kara. But that doesn't mean I don't want to be here.

The highs can be so high. And the lows? Heart wrenching.

On the day when Kara found a new medicine that worked, not only was she up and busy around the house, but she rode along to school to pick up her kids. She was able to see so many moms, so many friends she hadn't seen in ages.

Suddenly she was back and we had our girl again. Everyone swirled around her car at school like paparazzi. I stood to the side and laughed, snapping a few photos, surprised by a joy I hadn't felt in ages.

It felt so good to be happy that day, seeing her out and about, hugging the moms she loves who miss her so dearly.

The journey of walking through hard has amazingly good days mixed with unfathomably hard. Doing the heights and depths together is entering further in than perhaps you ever thought you would. A tentative first step becomes a leap, and suddenly you look back at those beginning shuffles and wonder how it came to this. All this heartbreak and beauty intermingled. Those two words shouldn't go together, but somehow, in this journey, they do.

Somehow, grace rises out of the ashes.

Alison is Kara's neighbor, and they met in the aftermath of a fire that ravaged Colorado Springs and consumed many homes. They had been evacuated, but fortunately their houses did not burn. When they returned to their neighborhood, their lives entwined.

I remember reading on Kara's blog about when she met Alison—
her neighbor with the young son who had cancer.

Not the kind of story I easily forget.

Alison learned her son had cancer when he was just shy of two
years old, and they were told the treatment would be surgery.

On the day she sat at the hospital waiting to see his doctor, a
friend who worked in the building texted her. *"I'm bringing you a
coffee."* It was a simple, sweet gesture. Her friend arrived, and they
were sitting together when the doctor came into the room.

He informed Alison that instead of just the surgery they'd
expected, her son was going to need a year of chemotherapy
treatment.

Alison says in that moment, she and her friend trauma-bonded.
Receiving that news together changed something between them.
This woman became the friend who showed up consistently—a per-
son who simply did instead of asking.

Alison remembers the friends who just did things. Dropped off
meals. Picked up her older son from school, often covering for her
at the last minute.

Two women who hadn't been lifelong friends with her still
entered the fray. They didn't let fear or lack of time invested in relationship stop them from showing up over and over again.

Alison has an understanding and a perspective of the heights and
depths met together that most of us don't have. She's been on both
sides. She's been the person suffering as the mother of a young boy
with cancer. The one trying to keep her older son's life as normal as
possible while driving the same streets week after week to the hospital for her younger son's treatment.

Alison met Kara as her son was finishing treatment and Kara was starting hers.

If anyone had an excuse to not show up, to heal, to rest, it was her. If anyone deserved to not hear the word "cancer" for a year, it was Alison. She could have called a time-out and said, "I'm weary. Not right now. Not yet." No one would have blamed her.

But she didn't choose the path of hiding away.

She showed up for Kara. She took the lessons she'd learned about community in her own hard and started doing them in another's life.

She sees where our world is lacking in community, and she shows up for those around her. She supplies the meal. Keeps the Tippetts freezer supplied with scones that disappear. Takes the kids. Is a friend.

As with each friend I've spoken with about this book, Alison admits her own sadness over losing Kara in the future. Near, far, every friend I've heard from has quietly uttered this same thought.

We feel selfish saying the words, but at the same time, they are true.

Losing Kara will leave a gaping hole in a different way in each person's life, and we're going to miss her. It's not about us, but at times we can't help uttering the sentiment that it feels as though it is.

Some suffering you'll walk through with others won't be this intense. Hopefully your person isn't facing a terminal illness. Hopefully their hard has an end and a new beginning on this earth. But whatever you are walking through together, it's confusing to figure out how to continue living your own life while your person is suffering in theirs.

A few months ago I spent the night at the hospital with Kara. It was sort of like a sleepover—one with a lot of pain and vomiting, laughter and deep conversation. It was a strange combination. I spent much of the night praying silently, begging God for relief for Kara.

Outside the hospital windows was an amazing panoramic view of the Rocky Mountains filling the skyline. And beneath the majestic mountains sat a freeway.

That night, I remember thinking about the lights from the cars and houses. It seemed surreal that people were still out doing things. Didn't they know my friend was suffering? Shouldn't the world stop while Kara was in the hospital?

But it didn't.

People kept flying down the interstate, focused on where they wanted to go next, passing the person in front of them as though they were in a race.

And they were, I suppose. To get somewhere. Be someone. Please someone. I run the same race daily.

I stopped and stayed still that night. It's torturous to be still while your friend is suffering. I must have offered to rub Kara's legs, hips, feet, and hands so many times I probably drove her nuts. She *may* have said something about me being "such a Martha," but that part of the night is fuzzy.

The desire to fix in a society that tells us to constantly *do* is hard to ignore. Kara was gracious with my need to help, sometimes accepting, other times telling me it was okay to just be.

In the morning, Kara finally slept while I shed silent tears and watched the first hints of light touch the mountain range. Pink on gray. White snow blowing from the top of Pikes Peak. I kept think-ing, *If God can do that, He can handle this.* It might not be in my timing or the way I want it, but He certainly can.

I sank into the knowledge that the God who made that moun-tain range knew every soul going by. Every single house light was a person He wants to come to Him.

The wonder of that touched me. He *knows* Kara, knows that we are calling out to Him for her, and she is one of how many? And yet the God who created glorious Pikes Peak knows each one of us. Wants each one of us. Cares that Kara is in pain. Cares that you or your person is suffering. Cares, cares, cares.

The world wants to tell us that He doesn't. But as Kara has told us many times, suffering is not the absence of God's goodness.

Just like it did that night, the world continues to flow around us during suffering, and we're dragged along with it, trying to figure out how to keep doing normal when life feels anything but.

Kara's kids continue to grow and have birthdays. We continue to go on trips, to shop for clothes while thinking of our friend who will probably never go shopping or go on a trip again. I take that back. Knowing Kara, she's just determined and stubborn enough to still make a trip happen.

And even while our friend is dying, time clicks on. And that causes a confusion, a dissonance in life.

In a culture where people avoid talking about death, Kara has gently forced us to deal with her truth. She's been honest and open about it, and in turn, she's asked us to do the same.

We still hope and pray that her story will end differently or that there's a medicine that can extend her life, but we've had to take a hard look at what it means to continue walking with someone whose suffering will not end until heaven.

This means having some brutally honest conversations. It also means moments of not having a clue what to say. Tears. Anger. Every emotion seems to be fair game.

Jason has worked to give the kids a sense of normalcy—taking Lake to a football game, the girls to a father-daughter dance. In the midst of hard, he strives to find the moments of good and pursues them.

He sets boundaries, accepting help with the kids during the day but wanting to have them home at night. He drives to school. Puts the kids to bed. Preaches sermons.

Even for him, time doesn't stop.

We have to keep functioning during suffering when all we want to do is crawl back into bed and wail.

Many days this hard road makes me crabby. I snap at my children and husband and have to apologize and start over again the next day. Most days I'm filled with a sadness I don't know how to express.

My husband and I often have the same conversation. He'll ask me if I'm okay, and I'll say no.

"What's wrong? Is it that your friend is dying or something else?"

"My friend dying," I'll answer.

He'll hug me. We sigh because there is no fixing this suffering. It simply is. And then somehow we keep functioning.

Near and far, we all whisper the same phrase. *"I don't know how to do this."*

And yet we just keep trudging on, not allowed the luxury of stopping during this storm.

We're all not okay as we struggle through these tough days, but we're trying to be. We're trying to love our children and spouses and be kind when that feels like a word from a foreign language. We pack lunches and apologize for losing it one more time. We drive to school and work. We take vacations that are planned even though it feels like cheating on Kara. We sit with her. We laugh. We have conversations we can't believe we're having. Sometimes we leave and bawl. Sometimes we're simply numb. Funeral plans are made. Life plans are made. We spend days and nights thinking of nothing else. And yet, there are moments and even days we pretend this isn't happening. We strive to believe God has a plan in this that is better than the one we see or understand. We choose to believe He is good when the world tells us He's not.

We might not be okay, but at least we're not okay together.

This journey might harbor the lowest of the lows at times, and I might not understand all of God's plans while I'm on this earth, but I have no doubt He is with us in it.

I feel Him, even when I can't explain Him.

With Kara's suffering, we've been given a gift of a long good-bye. It's both a height and depth mixed into one. We're thankful for every moment with her—we'll take every minute she's got. Yet it's so painful to see her suffer.

Some people who have lost loved ones quickly—without a word, kiss, hug, or shared last moment—would give anything for these days we're having with Kara even though they are hard.

But others see the quick flying away to heaven as a gift. Their person goes in the blink of an eye, and there is no earthly suffering, at least not for the one who departs for heaven.

Saying good-bye is hard. But saying it over the course of months, years even, is a path littered with potential land mines.

If showing up is a dance, then a long good-bye is like a slow dance with a partner who easily steps on toes. There are so many opportunities for us to make mistakes, yet also so many moments to grab and hold on to.

We had one of those confusing instances recently.

A friend who had moved away from Colorado was back visiting Kara. Since we all knew her before she moved, we moms planned a time to get together at one of our houses. Kara was in pain and could rarely leave her house, so when our queen of social gatherings heard about our plans, she felt left out. Once we realized this, we discussed a new plan and ended up moving the coffee date to Kara's house with the understanding that she might sleep through it if she wasn't feeling well.

Thankfully Kara mentioned her desire to be included. If she hadn't said anything, we would never have known how she felt. While we have to figure out how to continue doing life while our person is suffering, we also don't want to exclude them during their hardship.

When Alison's son was sick, she would often see updates on Facebook of things her friends were doing, without her. She wasn't invited. People tend to stop inviting the suffering person. They assume they are unable to participate. But in the same way we're still living—still functioning through a strange normal—so are the ones suffering. Alison wanted to be invited, even if she couldn't go. I would want that invitation too.

If your person is unable to do everything they used to do, what can they still do? Can they ride along on a shopping trip? Could you hit the grocery store together? Watch a movie? Look for ways you can still involve them.

The other day, I invited Kara to ride with me on an errand. I wasn't sure if it was the right decision because I knew she hadn't been able to leave her bed for a number of days. She didn't answer right away, and then finally she did respond. *"I just can't. But thanks for still asking me. Keep asking."* I felt relieved that I hadn't offended her in asking.

Kara isn't ready to be counted out. She wants the invitation even if she has to say no. What is your person like? Would they rather stay home? Or are they wishing for a chance to get out of the house?

Showing a person they matter in the midst of their suffering is a gift you can give.

While there have been many lows on this journey, there have also been many highs. Birthdays celebrated. Concerts, dinners, breakfasts, and coffee dates enjoyed. Friendships grew from seeds into beautiful flowers. A community formed and flourished. Books were written and released. Kara's first book, *The Hardest Peace*, came out last year, and we made the most of that accomplishment.

There are many moments of laughter and friendship to be consumed together while walking through hard. Kara and Jason have kept their sense of humor, and it's made many days bearable to be able to laugh.

This feels like a small normal.

There are times I question whether we should be laughing. Things feel so dire, Kara's prognosis so heavy, that laughter feels misplaced. But we have to embrace the glimpses of joy—and laughter—when we can. Don't let these slip away in the face of hard.

Tears will come easily, and they won't ask for permission. But the pockets of friendship we still get to have with Kara are part of the beauty in suffering.

When good moments come, cherish them. When there's something to celebrate, turn up the music and dance. Suffering gives us all the more reason to find the smallest good and expand on it.

And when the lows come, as they inevitably will, cry and weep and mourn. The sadness is just as important as the celebrating. Just as important.

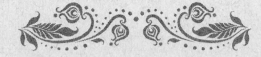

Kara

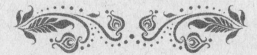

The long good-bye. Cancer has afforded me that, and I have tried to live faithfully in light of that dark gift. Never, at the age of thirty-eight, did I expect to be living under such fearsome blow after fearsome blow with each new diagnosis flattening us out. It is hard to recover to intentional living after each painful reminder of the limit on my days.

For my children, I have written blog posts, made videos, taped events, smiled and smiled into the camera to say, *"I was here with you, and it was beautiful."* The kids will one day see it as the long good-bye that it is. But right now they are simply the receivers of all the big love I have to give. Each day I fight the limitations this disease has placed upon me to love my children. It should not have taken cancer to cause me to abound in more and more love, but that is what Jesus chose to use to prompt my heart to extend the borders of me to love my people with more love than I could have otherwise known. I would have likely protected myself, lived safe, comfortable. But the long good-bye brings an amazing and seemingly senseless sharing of love.

With friends, moments are treasured up, stories shared, and questions asked. *"Will you? Will you love my people in my absence? You are not me, but will you try?" "Will you risk the effort to love my offspring with the love you have for your own children? I know it won't be the same, but will you try?" "Will you be there to help them shave their legs, navigate friendships, and struggle with relationships?"* The long good-bye allows me the time to ask specific questions like these of my friends.

With family, childhood memories come to the forefront of all conversation. As if to say, *"Remember, Kara? Remember this and take it with you. We shared life together, and it was a good life. Remember? We were there through it all, the triumph and the heartbreak. We were witness to it all."*

But with the long good-bye also comes the fear that something will be forgotten. Perhaps something left unsaid, undone, unresolved, and you fight to live your next moments well, hoping that grace will be present to help us all through the coming hard steps. The steps ahead, like those behind, that leave us uncertain.

In all this long good-bye, there is endless imagination that is taking place about what is, what will become, what might be. The long good-bye leaves me with the ability to bless Jason with the freedom to love again. He doesn't like that conversation. But it must happen. The long good-bye is filled with highs and lows, celebration and sadness. They are both equally important.

1. Romans 12:15 reads like this: "Rejoice with those who rejoice; mourn with those who mourn." There it is, right there in Scripture, a call to enter into both the joy and the sorrow. Showing up for someone in suffering will always mean that sorrow is in the room. But what can you do to celebrate the joy, even if it's a small joy? There is no handbook here, no recipe we can share with you. This is where you, and hopefully your community, can get creative, throw caution out the window, and stumble into some joy. Don't wait for things to get better. They may not.

2. Unless there is a sudden end to their suffering, we lose loved ones and friends a little at a time, pieces here, pieces there. Have you experienced this? How have you honored your person as pieces of them slip away? There are many ways to do this, but they all involve some variation of words: speak them, write them down, text them. To let the loss pass and not honor it in some way with words is to let silence have the last word.

Chapter 8

The Future Plans

There is a part of me that is screaming, much like Kara I think, We're not done yet.

We had a moment today. A moment when we were just two girlfriends talking about writing. It was small, short. But I walked away thinking, No, not yet.

Kara has entered this thing called hospice. It sounds like a black hole. It's not. It's a gateway to heaven; I get that. But will I ever be ready to let her go?

The idea that one day she won't be here to answer a text or dream big with me is ... unfathomable. I'm supposed to be mourning her. But how do you mourn someone who's still alive?

How do you walk the balance between learning to function without someone and gripping them so tightly that they can never break free?

I don't know how to let Kara go.

And truthfully I'm not supposed to yet. She's still here.

As long as there's a breath in her body, we will laugh. We will talk like girlfriends. We will live. She will live.

She's not done yet.

She has said there are corners slipping away from her. I want to gather them up and hold them for her. I'm numb. And when I'm not numb, I'm in shock. And when I'm not in shock, I'm crying.

How do you live while your friend is dying?

You go on loving your family. You hug your husband. You still laugh. You catch yourself, wonder if you should be laughing, and then laugh some more. Because yes, we all have to keep living. Even Kara, in this new hard. She has to keep living. She may not be fighting with chemo and radiation, but she is fighting.

She's fighting for a new normal.

One day, she's going to come out on the other side. A beautiful, pain-free, sunshine, farms-with-chickens kind of side. I believe that God is going to meet her there and kiss away her tears. I believe her pain will be gone and her joy will be unspeakable. That the God she's continued to worship even when Job-like tribulations and suffering have surrounded her will be waiting for her.

Can you imagine His face? Can you imagine His joy at seeing this child of His who would not forsake Him? How many small things have I questioned Him about? How many things did I try to tell God were deal breakers, as if I were in charge and not Him?

But not Kara.

She's been shouting His name. She's been proclaiming Him GOD. Not a sometimes Father, but an always Father. How many people have been changed because of her faith? Too many to count.

But before that heavenly joy for Kara, we stumble through hospice together.

We're all left in limbo. No. Limbo is too nice of a word. This is a tension, a grating of not knowing.

Will this be the last time I kiss her bald head? Do I say good-bye this time? Or do we simply talk like girlfriends, discussing our lives as though one of us isn't leaving?

Is there a right way to die?

I can only say this. My friend has LIVED well. Therefore her dying will be done well too.

───

I've been avoiding this chapter.

My tantrum was done quietly, stealth-like. I wrote other places, but when I came here, I couldn't fathom writing these words.

I don't want to write about the stark reality of my friend leaving this earth, the future, or what it will look like for her friends to mother her children.

Those subjects are not high on my happy list.

Tears fall instantly with this one. Other places in this book felt logical, especially when figuring out the best ways to show up for each other.

But this subject just feels like hurt, and I don't like it.

Kara once told me that the people who remained close to her were the people who accepted that she was dying. I wasn't that person for a long, long time. I fought believing that she was dying. I just couldn't accept it. Finally, I came to terms with that knowledge, though it felt like stepping barefoot across jagged glass.

Fine! I would huff. *I see it happening, but I'm still not okay with it.* But despite my adept skill at throwing tantrums, life doesn't always work the way we'd like it to.

Blythe is a dear friend of Kara's—and now mine. That's how this showing up thing works. I've stolen all of Kara's wonderful friends. She's a good picker, that Kara.

When Blythe was only twenty years old and still in college, she lost her parents in a car accident. Her journey with suffering started young, and she encountered amazing people showing up for her and people whose attempts were sorely lacking.

When she went back to school after her parents' deaths, she was greeted by another student there who told her she understood how Blythe felt. She, too, had endured hardship because her boyfriend had just broken up with her.

While this might seem outrageous to us, hurtful comments in response to suffering happen so often, even affecting Blythe's younger siblings who were still in school at the time.

Blythe prays over things like this for Kara and Jason's children— that they'll be protected from wounding things being said to them in the future.

When most of us couldn't handle conversations about dying, Blythe became Kara's safe place. She is the one Kara goes to when she needs to be reminded that her kids are going to make it without her. That they have the potential to turn out as wonderful as Blythe—one of the wisest and wittiest people I know.

Blythe even helped Kara plan her funeral so that Jason would be spared those details.

After speaking with Blythe about this, I could quickly see why she was the obvious choice. She lives with an eternity mentality. Heaven is not some far-off place for her. She believes it's just around the corner and even talks with her young children about heaven in everyday conversation.

In Blythe's presence, there is peace, joy, and expectation over our eternal home. She is both open and wise. Not afraid to talk about things that would make me cower under a rock. At least the old me. The new me that's getting more comfortable with my uncomfortable might stay within listening range so I can gain from her wisdom.

She and Kara have worked many, many hours together on details pertaining to the time when Kara's gone. They've worked out lodging for out-of-town guests who will come to the funeral, and they've planned the service itself. People have been asked to shop for clothes for the children in the year after Kara's gone. Others have been chosen to pursue the kids and become a safe place for them.

There is a plan to continue providing lunches and dinners for a year, and people have been designated to help with the housework (housekeeping and laundry). They've organized thank-you notes, printing them now so they are ready when needed. Someone is in charge of keeping track of who gives to the kids' trust funds, while Blythe is in charge of thank-you notes.

The list of what they've planned is long.

I used to wonder how Kara could deal with all these details, but then I realized her actions stem from selflessness.

Some people know they are going to die for days, weeks, or even years, and yet they do nothing to prepare for it. Kara has worked hard not only to be open and honest about dying but also to plan future moments of love for her family.

She sits in her bed, gazing upon photographs of four radiant faces hanging in frames on the wall, and she prays for her children's futures. Those prayers will live on long after she's gone from this earth. She's made videos for all the children in which she asks them questions about their future weddings. She's written birthday cards. Letters. Blogs. Books. Kara has loved her children and husband well into the future. And in choosing to talk about dying and working to plan what comes next, she's given her family a gift.

If she were selfish, she wouldn't deal with this harsh reality. But she pushes through the pain of her family's future without her in order to accomplish planning many things that will bless them in the future.

She reminds us girlfriends that one day Jason will remarry, and she expects us to welcome this "beautiful intruder." That's such a Kara-ism I had to keep the words as hers.

It's hard to imagine a future without her, but we know Kara's heart. We know that to honor her, we'll honor the choices Jason makes.

I was in another state visiting family when I got a text from Kara asking me if I was willing to do a certain job after she's gone. My daughter and I had just run to the store for something, and we sat in the grocery parking lot while I answered Kara, tears streaming down my face.

What I wanted to say was, *"I don't want to."* Not because I don't want to help, but because I don't want her to be dying. I don't want her to be planning a funeral with Blythe and passing out chores for a future without her.

But what I said was, *"Of course."*

In that moment and text conversation, her dying became far too real.

Many times Kara has spoken to us about taking a mothering role in her children's lives after she's gone. There is an understanding and a commitment from us to come alongside the kids, to fill in the places we can with a mother's love.

At times I wonder how we'll accomplish this—what it will look like. But then I'm reminded that Kara started letting us into her children's lives even during her first round of chemo.

She was much more able at that point, having times she could function during treatment, but I remember her letting go, not necessarily taking a step back from her kids but letting us mothers take a step toward them.

We joined forces. Kara was still in charge, but she made a decision to let us in.

Over the years, different moms have filled the role of caretaker—especially of her youngest—during different seasons. Kara's given grace to each one of these women. She trusts our mothering, our love for her children, and she doesn't haggle over small details that don't matter in the grand scheme of life. Just as she's worked to be a gracious receiver, she's also accepting of how we enter her children's lives.

She put her trust in God—and in the mothers around her—early on.

None of us expected that those beginning steps would turn into this. During that first year of cancer, we thought it would be only a short time that we'd be entering her kids' lives. Once she moved past her cancer battle, we thought our help would no longer be needed in the same way.

But that was not the story to be written.

And so things changed once again. Our roles as mothers have increased over the last year, months, even weeks, as more pieces of Kara slip away from us.

She's still with us, yet she's already not able to do many of the things she wants to do.

Kara has been preparing us for this all along. She's been paving this path for all of us. And now the fruits of that are evident in children who know us, who are comfortable with us. Her kids aren't going to be surprised by the moms in their life because we've already been there. Maybe not in the capacity we will one day be, but enough that we are safe for them.

Kara has always had a special gift in the area of motherhood. I've never seen someone delight in mothering the way she does. She truly enjoys her children and sees her role as a mom as a privilege, when so many of us see it as a job. One friend put it this way: *"The rest of us are trying to get through motherhood. Kara is in it."*

This beautiful quote perfectly describes our friend. While I sometimes see a day with kids as something to get through, she sees it as a privilege to come alongside her children and love them. To be kind to them. She enjoys them, yet she still disciplines.

Her mothering is an example of what we strive for in our own lives and what we hope to be for her children. Kind. Loving. Soft places to land on hard days. We'll never replace her, but we are ready to surround Jason and walk a new hard with him.

At times, those same sentiments I had at the beginning of this journey flare up again. How will I know what to do and how to help? What if I mess up or say the wrong thing?

There will be many, many of Kara's girlfriends who will surround her kids, and most likely, none of us have walked this path before. Certainly not this particular one.

But we'll still do it.

We already know that it simply starts with a step.

Justine has become a caretaker of the children in recent months. Their kids match in ages, and she's willingly stepped into this role. I think Justine would give up a kidney for someone she didn't know, yet when I asked her if child care would be her first instinctual way to help, she laughed and said no.

Though taking care of children wasn't on her radar, she says she finds such joy in watching Kara's children. God has given her a heart for this journey He's asked her to walk.

Watching her, I'm amazed by how she's meeting these children in love. Her heart is so tender. Since Kara is still with us, Justine works to be open if the children need to talk but accepts that they might not be ready. She doesn't push, but she does ask.

She gives out hugs and cuddles as much as she can. She's simply there, doing her best to love the kids through a hard we can't begin to fathom.

In the morning when I'm waking my children and at night when I'm putting them to bed is when I most often think of Kara and her kids. Those moments of quiet mothering break my heart into shattered pieces. I know Jason will be there. I know he'll love the kids and be gentle with them. But they will miss their mother with an ache that brings me to tears.

We mothers will come around the kids and smother them with love, but I can't help questioning whether we'll be enough.

Is there enough mother between all of us to make this better?

No. There isn't. But with God, there will be.

He loves the motherless and the orphans. He will hold them close and fill the gaps. He is the whole of the comfort, and we, as mothers, are just tools, privileged to be an extension of the community He's planned for us to be.

Recently, Kara's dream of making it to the beach happened. And while she and Jason ran away together for a few short nights, different families took their kids and planned fun activities to fill their weekend.

The night we had the kids, we were driving home when their laughter and chatter filled the car. A rush of moisture filled my eyes. *Is this what it will be like when she's gone?*

The thought felt wrong, as though I'm waiting for her to leave this earth. But I'm not. I don't want her to go. Ever. But these moments feel like glimpses into a time without her.

One child rolls her eyes and tries to hide her smile when my husband teases her. Another simply feels comfortable wherever she goes. The whole of them are loud and boisterous, finding joy in these moments even though heartache looms.

This all started long ago, I think.

And I'm thankful.

Isn't that the strangest emotion? I'm fighting tears and smiling at the same time while we drive through a darkened town, the streetlights shining down on a vehicle full of noise and life. I'm so thankful Kara's let us be a part of her children's lives.

She's giving *us* a gift. We're the ones who are blessed.

It happened to be Valentine's Day, and my husband and I didn't think about missing a fancy dinner with each other. Our dinner was a bunch of kids being kids, running and squirreling around when they should be sitting down to eat. Just being kids.

And I'm so thankful for those moments.

I don't know what all of this is going to look like after Kara's gone. I don't know if the kids will act as though everything is okay but be broken inside. I don't know if they'll allow us to hold them while they cry, or if all of that will be reserved for Jason.

I only know we're willing. We're here. And that God will meet us there.

Kara

Here is one thing I know to be true. My children will never be motherless. Not one day. No, my children have a swarm of mothers surrounding them who will fiercely love and protect them throughout their days. Though I, their first mother, will be gone, they will remain well mothered the rest of their days. We have fought for this reality for our children. We have opened wide our stories to people we love in hopes that they would take seriously their call to covenant living with our children after I breathe my last. I see a growing heart commitment in my friends for just that kind of living.

How did I get there? That is the question. How did I invite so many women into my life to make this a reality? Well, part necessity, part personality. I needed to, and my personality longs to raise my children in a village, not on an island. So before I was dying, I was living large in community. I always thought I would be the one to be asked to one day help mother another. But no, I'm the one asking. It's not a simple thing to ask, as I already know the crushing burdens so many families live under. To ask them also to partner with me in parenting my children seems a tall order to ask of any friend.

My children will keenly feel the absence of me, their specific mama, but they will know mama love from so many corners of life it will be beautiful to behold. It's the best of living in community. From the outset of my diagnosis, we have invited community in, knowing we would have needs that would go out to our community.

As a mama, it's hard to open my hand to this story—the story that I may not be the only mama known to my children. But I will be the first mama known to my babies. That matters; that is what I get. And in my absence, my dearest community of girlfriends will lend their strength to our weakness and need.

I am not naive. I know some of the mothering responsibility will fall to our oldest daughter. Eleanor was born a nurturer, and she cares well for her younger brother and sisters. I have often had to remind her to be a sister, not a mother. Still, I know she will carry a heavier load with her siblings—helping them navigate hard waters without a mama.

Jason will also have a heavy weight of widowerhood placed on his already weary shoulders. But sufficient grace will be present. I believe that with everything that is in me. He will have to ask our friends for help when needs arise. He will surely stumble as he learns to be alone. I cannot imagine his role, but rarely do I despair the sense of my children being without mothering. Mothering is an action I see being taken seriously by many I love dearly. So, will my children be mothered well? Yes. And what about Jason? Pray for him, please. I often tell my girlfriends that this is going to be Jason's *Job* moment. That God is going to redeem this hard for him. I know he won't be to that point for a long while after I'm gone. I know his tender heart will be bruised beyond comprehension. But when he is ready, I expect grace upon grace for him. She will be a beautiful intruder.

1. What's your hard? Remember, hard is hard. Cancer, loneliness—one does not trump the other. There is another kind of showing up that we've talked about but not phrased in this way yet. It's *showing up for yourself*, and that happens by asking for help. It's what Kara has done all along the way, setting aside whatever pride or independence might have been there, and saying, "Help me." Showing up for herself in this way has been the doorway that each of her friends has been invited to walk through. So, what is your hard? And how can you show up for yourself in that? Whom can you ask to help you? What might you ask them for?

2. We try to teach our children so many things. At some point along the way we realize most of what they learn is from watching us—how we speak, how we behave, how we spend our time and money. Showing up for someone in suffering is a way to pass on to the next generation one of the most beautiful and beneficial lessons there is about life. It may be your children who see it, or it may be your spouse or another friend or church member or neighbor. Your showing up will make an impression on them. It may lead them to imitate your big love in the life of someone else who is suffering. Showing up is being a witness to the God who cares, the God who is with us to the very end and beyond. How has witnessing others showing up had an impact on you?

Chapter 9

The Beauty of Community

I imagine there will be a garden in heaven tended by a beautiful woman. Her beauty will radiate from the inside, just like it did on earth. There will be a farm-house with chickens and a wide porch. Many chairs to sit and rock and share in.

I believe Kara's community in heaven will be mag-nificent. I imagine the members—ones from all corners of the earth—will recognize each other without introduction. There will be joy and laughter. Hugs and rejoicing. And none of the pain and suffering that has joined us together on this earth will remain.

Kara will probably still cook dinner for anyone who wants to come over. And maybe even offer beer or a glass of wine. Which means we'll probably all be sent to the still-slightly-sinner side of heaven—the one that plays loud music and believes in dancing.

I imagine her house will have a beach next to it with waves lapping against the shore.

One day, her children will meet her in that garden just like her Savior did.

But before that day so far away that will feel like only moments, her children will grow up wise

and strong, compassionate and beautiful of heart. I believe God has big plans for them. I believe Jason will weep, and our God will hold him through it.
I believe.

In the beginning of her cancer journey—before she'd lost any hair—Kara had planned a photo shoot to capture her family together. A friend was over, and Kara commented on the fact that she didn't know what to wear and that she liked this friend's dress.

Without pause, the friend gave it to Kara to keep.

Kara began calling it her grace dress. She wore it many times to many hard appointments—her reminder of God showing up.

Throughout her fight with cancer, Kara has always looked for these moments—and, even on these very hard days, is still looking for them. She believes grace always shows up.

On particularly tough days, I would wonder if grace was going to appear. I would question God. *Where are You in this? Show us, please.*

And He did. Over and over again.

Though it wasn't always in the ways I expected it or in the answers I wanted, He always showed up. Often, grace was found in the small things. When we're looking only for the big things that knock us over, we're missing the small graces.

We may not be able to tangibly touch all the ways God shows up, but we can feel Him. We can trust Him. And we know He's with us.

And though our peace is mixed strongly with sorrow, it's still present.

Kara's hospital bed recently arrived at their house. It's been more than two months since she first entered hospice care, and we've had more days with her than some of us expected at the beginning of this. Yet at the same time, fewer days than we want.

We tend to get greedy with Kara's days.

Even now, as she wrote on her blog, she's still looking to Him:

> I feel too young to be in this battle, but maybe I'm not in a battle at all. Maybe I'm on a journey, and the journey is more beautiful than any of us can comprehend. And if we did understand, we would hold very loosely to one another because I'm going to be with Jesus. There is grace that will seep into all the cracks and pained places when we don't understand. In the places we don't understand we get to seek. And how lovely is one seeking truth. Stunning.

Heaven is greater than anything I could ever imagine, and while I don't want the world to go on without Kara, I want that joy for her. I want her pain to go away. I want her mind to be free again to worship, write, and glory in a God she never denied.

And because of the gift of our beautiful Savior, I believe that we'll meet again one day. I believe that relationships will be restored and will be even more beautiful than they were on earth. I think about how in heaven we'll be able to completely skip the chapter in this book on insecurity. Thank goodness.

And then I realize none of these words will make sense there. There will be no place for talking about suffering because it will be a foreign concept to us.

I never used to dream about heaven. But walking through suffering with Kara has changed that for me. Now, my soul whispers, *Jesus, come.*

I long for a new earth. For the absence of these hurts.

Today, I'm going to see Kara. We have a schedule now. Short increments of time when we get to spend a few moments with her.

She's fading.

And oh. My. Soul. It. Is. Hard.

Again, I question if this is the last time I'll see her. But I have the promise that it's not. One day. One day I'm going to sit on that porch with my friend again.

And what a glorious day that will be.

The concept of showing up can feel so broad, so overwhelming, and yet look where it brought us. The community God has made in the midst of this horrible hard is beautiful to see. It stretches across seas and oceans, languages and age. Kara writes a blog post and so many answer. I see their pain. It's the same as ours here. It doesn't matter that they haven't met Kara. They know her because she's let them know her. They've entered in with her. With all of us.

In the beginning of writing this book, I wondered how this community that loves Kara would accept me, would accept us writing this book together. *They don't want you. You're not Kara.* The whispers stole words from me until I realized something.

This community isn't about Kara. It's about Christ.

And it's breathtaking. We have held each other up and will continue to hold each other up. I believe it will be quite the commotion when this group meets in heaven one day.

When I look around at the community that was born during this suffering, I see so many, many people who weren't there and blessings that didn't exist before Kara's cancer. And while I'd gladly trade in this disease for an easier road for my friend—for everyone around her—I see the beauty God has orchestrated.

As I interviewed friends for this book, I would often ask them a question: *"What's your hard?"*

We all have suffering in our lives. It might not be to the extent of Kara's, but we each have our own battle, our own hard path we've been asked to walk.

One friend didn't give the answer I expected to that question. Her husband travels frequently, often for weeks at a time, to work with orphans in other countries. It's a lot of work for her when he's gone because they have three kids and she works part-time.

I questioned her. *"Isn't that your hard?"*

She nodded, but then quickly went on to explain: *"But I don't think of it that way because God has redeemed that hard. He's made something beautiful from it."*

Those words struck me and stayed with me throughout this whole book.

God asked this friend to walk a certain path, and she's obeyed. In that, she has been blessed, redeemed, kept.

The hard we've walked with Kara has also been redeemed in this way. In the brightest and darkest moments, God has been with us through it and will continue to be.

If God asks us to do something, then He's also going to show up to carry us through it. And when we walk in community with one another, we will be kept.

When I think of the girlfriends, the relationships that have formed during this suffering, my eyes fill with tears. These women have become a community like no other—a place to cry and hug, tender hearts who understand each other in amazing ways.

When I've been stuck in knowing how best to represent these women or this community as I write, they are the ones I go to. They remind me of the good in this journey. The story of these friendships is beautiful to behold.

If you are around the moms near Kara, you'll hear a phrase used when we greet each other: *"Hey, mama."*

It's another Kara-ism. Something she says when she sees us, and a greeting we now use with each other.

Mama has become a term of endearment. A code. Sorrow and joy are wrapped up in that one word.

It's an example of one of the fruits of this community. It might sound small, but it is mighty. It's a glimpse of something that didn't exist before but that now has its own heartbeat and meaning. Friend. Wife. Mother. Safe place.

Community builds this.

Showing up has its own language, its own culture. Joy unspeakable. Pain unbearable. These two emotions are intermingled in this journey of beautiful hard.

The fruits that have bloomed from the labor of showing up are many. Soft hearts. Relationships formed. Lives changed. Faith gained.

And showing up has spread like a ripple effect, influencing circle after circle. During hard times, all of us surrounding Kara have had people show up for us. It might be by text message, note, card, flowers, a meal, or just the reminder that someone is praying not only for Kara but for us.

We all cling to those moments and prayers.

One friend mentioned that an acquaintance of hers started messaging her to check in and say she was praying for her. This thoughtfulness almost always coincided with a hard day or a day that she'd seen Kara. When we follow the prompting of the Holy Spirit, He uses us as vessels for Him to show up.

Other friends mentioned that a girlfriend has shown up for them by bringing meals and always checking on them and praying for them. She's a support to them even though she doesn't personally know Kara. This woman has shown up beautifully for her friends—a testament that will live on long after this time of suffering.

There are also many silent supporters who make it possible for people to show up. The husbands, grandparents, and friends who come alongside each of us are a huge part of what makes this possible. Many husbands drop off meals. Many children have been watched by fathers and grandparents so that moms can show up for Kara.

As I'm writing, I just received a text that said my friend is praying for me today—for these words that are tapping from my fingertips.

The beauty in all of this is that this isn't my story. This isn't even Kara's story.

This is *our* story. The story of a community that grew from ashes and has become a beautiful thing to behold. Not by our strength—if anything, it was by our weaknesses.

It's the story of suffering being redeemed. Of God showing up in the midst of community here on earth.

The Mundane Faithfulness community that's been built online is another example of the fruits of showing up. So many Christian authors face judgments and even harsh words from online communities. But that seems to be absent from this one. I've often wondered about this as I read the comments from people who are invested in Kara's journey.

There is grace in this community. Platitudes are not offered. There's no "God won't give you more than you can handle" comments. So many have come to Mundane Faithfulness while in their own place of suffering. Sorrow and stories are shared and accepted for the painful things they are. There's no shouting. No judging. People honor one another in this group in a way that's beautiful to see. They show up with words and prayers, even if it's through a computer screen.

In our culture, we don't often see community done the way Kara has modeled it for us. And when we do, something in us whispers, *I want that.*

Mickey has been a mentor in Kara's life and another example of the beauty in suffering. Before this—without this trial—we wouldn't have known this wonderful, wise woman. But now we do. And we've all gained insight from her. We all agree that we want to be Mickey when we grow up.

We were speaking about Kara's gift in growing community when Mickey mentioned that most of us have never seen good friendships done well. Especially between women. So often there's jealousy and cattiness.

We aren't showing and teaching young girls how to do community together. Because of this, more women grow up not knowing how to enter safely in with one another.

When we see Kara and the community she's built, we want to join in, to be a part of it. But Mickey advises that we should look at what Kara's modeling, then go out and do that in our own circles.

Can you imagine the influence on the world?

Kara has given us a legacy, one we can take and apply in our own lives and our own communities. One that will live on long after her last breath.

The other day someone offered to fill a need for Jason and Kara, and Jason was able to respond that they didn't need that particular help. Their community has become so big and amazing that he was able to say, "Thank you, but we're okay." He asked them to take that gift, that love, and go out and serve someone else in need.

At the moment I write this, our girl is holding on, but her grip on this place is loosening. Jesus wants His Kara. And we're all going to have to figure out how to do this without her.

Once again, I want to say I don't know how. And once again, those words might be true.

But He knows the next step, even when we don't. Just as He's been there for every stumble of this journey, He'll be there for the next too.

Dear Kara,

Above all else—above cancer and suffering and the family we've pledged to love with all our mothering pooled into one—you are quite simply a friend.

To say that we're going to miss you would be like saying we'd miss the sun if it didn't come up in the morning.

I can promise you this. We will love your family. And when the next thing comes, we will stumble through that together too.

Because you taught us well how to enter in with one another.

You taught us to show up.

Kara

I don't want this to end. The book, and my life. I'm not afraid of dying; it's just that I don't want to go. But just like I've tried to show up for life, I'll show up for death. I am ready.

If there is one constant in our world, it's pain and suffering. Just look around. It might be a woman dying of cancer. It might be a neighbor dying inside of loneliness. We have to be careful not to put a grade on pain, like hers is greater than his. Pain is pain, and suffering is suffering. What this means, though, is that each and every day of our lives is filled with opportunities to just show up in someone's life. We can set aside a little of ourselves, step into someone else's story, and see how Jesus shows up. And, my dear friends, Jesus always shows up. Always.

I use the word *community* a lot. I do that intentionally. It is a very important word to me. But I have to tell you that you could go back through everything I've said or written and every time you come across the word *community*, you could substitute the word *friend*. That's what Jill and I are talking about. Friends show up for each other. It may be some of the best work we do in our lives, being a friend.

It's kind of tough to write the last sentence of a book. I still want to say so much. My little body has grown tired of battle, and treatment is no longer helping. But what I see, what I know, what I have is Jesus. He has still given me breath, and with it I pray I would live well and fade well. By degrees doing both, living and dying, as I have moments left to live. I get to draw my people close, kiss them, and tenderly speak love over their lives. I get to pray into eternity my hopes and fears for the moments of my loves. I get to laugh and cry and wonder about heaven. I do not feel like I have the courage for this journey, but I have Jesus—and He will provide. He has given me so much to be grateful for, and that gratitude, that wonder about His love, will cover us all. And it will carry us—carry us in ways we cannot comprehend.

"Losing myself in the startling light of Kara's story, I have found who I am, who He is, and more of the meaning of every breath."

Ann Voskamp, *New York Times* bestselling author

finding grace in the everyday

Kara Tippetts knows the mundanity of life as a young mother, the joy of watching her children grow, and the devastating reality of stage-four cancer. In *The Hardest Peace*, she invites us to see the grace of the everyday in all seasons of life and to live well even when living is hard.

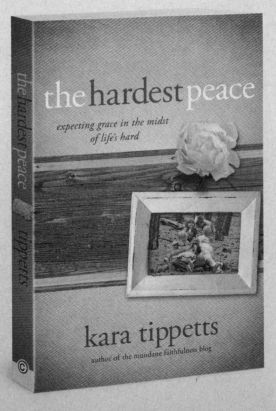

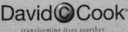